BLACK HEALTH
LIBRARY GUIDE

HEART DISEASE AND HYPERTENSION

BLACK HEALTH LIBRARY GUIDE

HEART DISEASE AND HYPERTENSION

Vital Health Information for
African Americans

Paul A. Jones, M.D.
with Angela Mitchell

Edited by Linda Villarosa
Nutritional Advisor, Maudene Nelson
Illustrated by Marcelo Oliver

KENSINGTON BOOKS
KENSINGTON PUBLISHING CORP.
http://www.kensingtonbooks.com

KENSINGTON BOOKS are published by

Kensington Publishing Corp.
850 Third Avenue
New York, NY 10022

First Kensington Printing: January, 2000
10 9 8 7 6 5 4 3 2 1

Printed in the United States of America

Contents

Introduction

The numbers are undeniable: despite great medical and technological advances since the 1960s, African-Americans are still suffering and dying from a host of ill-nesses at higher rates and at younger ages than whites. The average black American enjoys about fifty-six years of healthy life, compared to sixty-four years for whites. Our infant mortality rate is falling, but it's still twice as high as for white women. For every thirteen cancer deaths among whites, there are seventeen deaths among blacks. We face twenty-four cases of tuberculosis for every 9 white cases.

We are less likely to have health insurance, less likely to receive health care services, and less likely to feel that our doctors really care about our health. Recent studies have demonstrated that even when we do access health care, we don't receive certain treatments as frequently as whites. "When you take black and white Americans and exactly the same situation, like being hospitalized for a heart attack and having the same insurance, the chance that the black patient will get the advanced care is much less than it is for the white patient," says Sara Rosen-baum, director of the Center for Health Policy Research at George Washington University. "The medical system appears to treat them differently."

Many of the differences in the disease rates, mortality rates, and rates of treatment also reflect black/white disparities in income and education, and the fact that those with better insurance or more money are more likely to access the best care because they can pay for it.

These explanations are only part of the story, however. Even African-Americans with college educations and good jobs suffer disproportionately from a number of illnesses. We know that discrimination places a daily and heavy stress on us, and this stress, over time, is causing much unnecessary suffering and early death. Obviously, discrimination has not been eliminated from the health care system, and it is unlikely that this will happen quickly.

But there is still more to the problem of our failing collective health. Many of us don't take care of ourselves as well as we should. Chances are you know a woman who keeps putting off a mammogram because she's too busy or a heavy smoker who says he won't quit because he believes "you've got to die of something." While it is true that jobs and families demand tremendous amounts of time, everyone needs to make time to take care of themselves. An annual visit to the doctor, even when you feel fine, is one thing everyone should take time for.

Of course, this isn't always easy. Some of us are cut out of the health care system because doctors' fees are exorbitant, we don't have health insurance, and there are few physicians in our communities. But this isn't the case for everyone. We often take chances with our health, eating foods we know aren't healthy, putting off exercise, and teaching our children these same bad habits. We may know that we are obese, or that the smoker's hack we've developed does not bode well for a healthy future. But we're only human, we tell ourselves. What's a little extra weight or another cigarette going to hurt?

Perhaps the biggest barrier to improving our health is a lack of education about disease and its prevention. This is true of hypertension, heart disease, cancer, AIDS, diabetes—you name it. Studies have shown that when people are aware of what effects their habits have on their health, they are more likely to make constructive change and stick with it. Education is the first step to prevention, and prevention is the way to reclaim our lives and our health. No amount of national health care insurance will make up for our lack of initiative in taking responsibility for our health. We all have the power to do it, and by reading this book, you are taking the first step toward a healthier future for you and your family.

Part I

Taking Control of Your Cardiovascular Health

CHAPTER 1

Calculating Your
Cardiovascular Risks

Where were you on November 25, 1987? If you're like most African-Americans, you were mourning the sudden loss of an extraordinary mayor, Harold Washington of Chicago, who died of a massive heart attack. Like millions of us, the mayor harbored several risk factors for cardiovascular disease: he led a fast-paced life, running from meeting to meeting, mediating strikes and city council wars, and staying up late to catch up on his reading. At 5 feet 10 inches and 265 pounds, he was more than 60 pounds overweight; he'd smoked for more than thirty years (although he'd claimed to have quit); and both his blood pressure and cholesterol levels were high. Had Mayor Washington taken control of his health, he may have survived to fight the good fight another day for the people of Chicago.

Needless to say, Mayor Washington was far from alone in suffering from cardiovascular disease or in ignoring its dangers long enough for it to kill him. Hypertension (high blood pressure) and coronary heart disease are two of the top health problems facing Americans today. According to the latest statistics released by the National High Blood Pressure Education Program in October 1992, an estimated 50 million Americans have high blood pressure and about 14 million have some degree of coronary artery disease. Every year, these conditions contribute to roughly 1.1 million heart attacks and 600,000 strokes; of these two numbers, nearly 640,000 of them are fatal.

Among African-Americans, cardiovascular disease is even more epidemic and problematic. Some recent studies estimate that as many as 35 percent of all African-American adults may have high blood pressure compared with about 22 percent of the adult white population. In addition, hypertension in black Americans tends to appear at an earlier age and is often not treated as aggressively as cases of hypertension in whites. Although the prevalence of coronary heart disease is similar among black and white Americans, a heart attack is more likely to be fatal in African-Americans.

Why is there such a disparity between blacks and whites when it comes to cardiovascular disease? As discussed in the Introduction, African-Americans continue to suffer from a profound lack of access to health insurance, health care, and health care education.

We are also less likely to receive certain medical procedures, such as angiography and bypass operations. Not only are doctors less likely to recommend such procedures because of racial discrimination and the perception that blacks are less able to pay, but blacks are more likely to refuse that type of care than are whites. Some blacks feel that doctors want to treat us as guinea pigs, testing new drugs and procedures on the least educated and least powerful among us. The fact that blacks make up just 3 percent of the physician population but about 12 percent of the general population only adds to the sense of alienation from modern medicine some blacks feel.

In addition, many of the risk factors for cardiovascular disease, which are described in detail below, are more common in the black community than in the white. A majority of black Americans tend to be salt-sensitive, for instance, which means that our blood pressure is more likely to be affected by the amount of salt we eat; this tendency appears to be far less pervasive in the white population. More African-Americans than white Americans smoke cigarettes, and more blacks than whites suffer from diabetes. These conditions also add to the likelihood that hypertension and/or heart disease will develop in a given individual.

Amid all this gloom and doom, however, there is some very good news for blacks and whites alike: hypertension and heart disease are among the most preventable and treatable conditions in all of medicine. Just one decade after the federal government created the National High Blood Pressure Education Program in 1972 to help stem the epidemic of cardiovascular disease, physicians estimated that about 8 million fewer Americans had hypertension and some 180,000 strokes and an even greater number of heart attacks had been prevented. Not only are drugs and surgical techniques more effective, but lifestyle factors, such as proper diet and sufficient exercise, are now recognized as life-saving strategies by more Americans—black and white—than ever before.

Without doubt—and I'll say this again and again throughout this book—knowledge is power when it comes to cardiovascular health. The very fact that you are reading this book is proof that taking care of your health has become a priority for you. Indeed, you've taken a very big step to make sure that your cardiovascular system stays in good working order.

RISK FACTORS FOR HYPERTENSION AND HEART DISEASE

Risk factors are those conditions and/or habits associated with the increased likelihood of developing a disease. Cigarette smoking, for instance, is a risk factor for the development of lung cancer because chemicals in smoke are known to affect lung tissue in a detrimental way. Hypertension itself is a risk factor for other cardiovascular diseases, including stroke and coronary heart disease (Table 1).

The likelihood that you, as an individual, will develop a certain disease is influenced by both *uncontrollable* and *controllable* risk factors. Someone with sickle cell anemia, for instance, inherited the disorder from his or her parents; obviously, the genetic factor that causes the disease to occur in this individual is uncontrollable.

Other risk factors, however, are controllable: by making certain changes in your lifestyle or by taking medication, you can help protect yourself from developing a certain disease. If you stop smoking, for instance, you have taken control over that risk factor for lung cancer (as well as for a host of other potentially lethal conditions, including high blood pressure and heart disease).

The quiz in Table 1 will help you to calculate your risks of developing cardiovascular disease. Keep in mind that this test is not meant to frighten you: even if you find that you have a moderate or even very high risk of developing cardiovascular disease, you should not consider yourself *doomed* to actually suffer from it. A high score simply indicates that you may be *more likely* to develop high blood pressure and/or heart disease than someone with low risk. By taking the quiz, you'll be able to determine what factors in your life may predispose you to developing hypertension and/or heart disease.

Calculating and Evaluating Your Score

30–45: Cardiac Red Alert Your score indicates that you are at very high risk for hypertension and/or heart disease. Not only do you have one or more uncontrollable risk factors—such as being black, being over forty, and/or having a family history of cardiovascular disease—but you also have several dietary and other habits that are adversely affecting your body. If you do not already know the status of your blood pressure and the health of your heart, I recommend that you see your physician immediately for an evaluation. In addition, it's

TABLE 1 Your Cardiovascular Self-Test

Uncontrollable Risk Factors

How old are you?
Under 40 (score 1 point)
40–55 (score 2 points)
Over 60 (score 3 points)   _____

Which sex are you?
Female (1 point)   Male (3 points)   _____

**Have any of your close relatives—mother, father, sister, brother,
   aunt, uncle—had a stroke or heart attack?**
No (1 point)
Yes, one relative (2 points)
Yes, more than one relative (3 points)   _____

Controllable Risk Factors

How often do you consume red meat and/or whole eggs?
Twice a week or less (1 point)
Three times a week (2 points)
More than three times a week (3 points)   _____

Do you smoke?
I have never smoked/I gave up smoking more than five years ago (1 point)
I gave up smoking less than five years ago (2 points)
I smoke ten or more cigarettes a day (3 points)   _____

Do you exercise on a regular basis?
I participate in vigorous exercise (running, cycling, swimming, etc.) at
   least three times a week (1 point)
I am active once or twice a week (2 points)
I lead a sedentary life (3 points)   _____

Are you overweight?
I am less than ten pounds overweight (1 point)
I am between ten and twenty pounds overweight (2 points)
I am more than twenty pounds overweight (3 points)   _____

Do you have a history of diabetes?
No (1 point)
Yes (3 points)   _____

TABLE 1 Your Cardiovascular Self-Test (cont.)

Do you add salt to food while cooking?
No (1 point)
Yes (3 points)   —

How often do you eat canned foods?
Less than three times a week (1 point)
Three times a week (2 points)
Every day (3 points)   —

Do you eat pork, especially salt pork, ham hocks, canned ham, bacon, or sausage, more than twice a week?
No (1 point)
Yes (3 points)   —

Do you regularly drink more than two alcoholic beverages a day?
No (1 point)
Yes (3 points)   —

Do you use any illegal drugs, particularly cocaine?
No (1 point)
Yes (3 points)   —

How do you react to stress?
I feel a sense of purpose when faced with a professional or personal challenge (1 point)
I feel that life is a constant struggle and sometimes feel frustrated and angry (2 points)
I feel trapped in a hard, sad, endless struggle against impossible odds (3 points)
                                                                        —

                                        YOUR TOTAL   —

---

up to you to take control of your health by eliminating as many of the controllable risk factors from your life as possible.

15–30: Warning If you're not careful, the food you eat and the lifestyle you lead may eventually cause your blood pressure to become elevated and your coronary arteries to develop atherosclerosis, especially if you've answered any of the first four "uncontrollable risk factor" questions in the affirmative. Make any changes to improve the health of your cardiovascular system as soon as possible to avoid the often devastating consequences of uncontrolled high blood pressure and heart disease.

14 or Below: Stay on Guard So far, you've managed to avoid many of the common pitfalls on the road to cardiovascular health, but it's important to keep yourself on track. Take a look at the controllable risk factors you feel apply to you and make it a priority to eliminate them from your life in order to maintain and improve your health.

Keep in mind that risk factors for cardiovascular disease are cumulative—the more that apply to you, the more likely you are to damage your heart and vessels. In other words, someone who smokes, has diabetes, and is obese has a much greater chance of developing hypertension and/or heart disease than a nonsmoking, nondiabetic person who needs to lose weight. The good news is that you can improve the health of your cardiovascular system by eliminating just one risk factor at a time.

UNDERSTANDING YOUR RISK FACTORS

Despite the multitude of warnings sounded by the media about the importance of preventing or arresting cardiovascular disease, literally millions of people suffer from high blood pressure and heart disease without realizing it. As stated above, many cases of cardiovascular disease are preventable—*if* you are willing to make changes in your diet, exercise, and other personal habits (Table 2). Let's take a look at each of the possible elements involved in cardiovascular disease, starting with the four uncontrollable risk factors: age, sex, family history, and race. Although they are beyond your control, it's important for you to understand the effect they may have on your health.

TABLE 2 Risk Factors for Cardiovascular Disease

Uncontrollable	Controllable
Age	High cholesterol
Sex	Cigarette smoking
Family history	Sedentary lifestyle
Race	Diabetes
	High salt intake
	Alcohol and drug abuse
	Stress

Uncontrollable Risk Factors

Age Growing older is both a blessing and a curse. Most of us say we would like to live long lives, but we usually add the word "healthy" to that statement. Many people fear that they will live to an advanced age but will be too ill to derive much pleasure from life. Indeed, there are certain aspects of aging that cannot be avoided: if we live long enough, for instance, we all will have wrinkles and our hair will turn gray or become thin.

Until recently, high blood pressure and even heart disease were considered inevitable side effects of the aging process. It is true that after decades of keeping your body nourished with oxygen-rich and nutrient-rich blood, your heart and blood vessels will show some signs of wear and tear. However, recent evidence proves that everyone can limit the damage by eliminating as many of the controllable risk factors involved in cardiovascular disease as possible. No matter how old you are, taking steps to reduce your risk of developing cardiovascular disease now will help ensure that you don't run into trouble later.

Sex Generally speaking, both black and white men suffer more hypertension and heart disease than their female counterparts. It is unclear exactly why this is true, but researchers believe that the female hormones, estrogen and progesterone, play an important role in protecting women from the ravages of atherosclerosis, a contributing factor to both hypertension and heart disease. It isn't until women are past the age of menopause, when female hormone levels decrease dramatically, that women have equal and even greater rates of high blood pressure and heart disease.

Indeed, cardiovascular disease in women is a serious health problem. Between the ages of forty-five and sixty-five, one in nine women has some form of cardiovascular disease and the percentage rises to one in three over the age of sixty-five. Perhaps most shockingly, of the approximately 500,000 fatal heart attacks per year, almost half occur in women and that number appears to be rising every year. Unfortunately, the reasons for the increase in cardiovascular disease in women are largely unknown because it is only in recent years that the scientific community has chosen to study women's health at all; for decades, women have been excluded from major studies.

The health of *black* women, then, has been especially affected by the bias toward white men in the medical research community. It is only in recent years that the frightening severity of cardiovascular disease in black women has begun to be universally recognized. The truth is that heart disease is the most common cause of death in black women ages thirty-five to seventy-four. At every age, black women are more than twice as likely as white women to have hypertension and/or heart disease. Although the incidence of cardiovascular disease increases after menopause among both black and white women, black women far more quickly surpass their white counterparts.

As you'll see below, the reason for the disparity in cardiovascular disease between black and white women may be because more black women than white women are obese and more black women than white women suffer from diabetes. Thanks to recent efforts by the National Institutes of Health and other major health organizations in the United States, more attention will be paid in the future to the health of women, both black and white.

Family History Perhaps you're reading this book because your parents or grandparents have hypertension and you're worried that you somehow inherited it from them. Can disease be passed down from generation to generation? Unfortunately, along with other traits like eye color and height, your parents may have passed on to you certain physical characteristics that may predispose you to developing hypertension and/or heart disease.

Indeed, scientists have determined that some people inherit a genetic *predisposition* to disease—in other words, those with one or more relatives with a certain disease are more likely to develop that disease than people who do not have such a family background. In some disorders, the genetic component is so strong that nothing can be done to alter the course of the disease. These diseases, such as sickle cell anemia, hemophilia, and cystic fibrosis, involve just one or two faulty genes and are relatively rare.

Most common adult diseases, including hypertension and heart disease, involve a multiple number of genes; for example, geneticists have identified nearly twenty genes that cause just one aspect of coronary heart disease. In addition, many of those genes express themselves differently depending on the circumstances. If a person has inherited a tendency to retain sodium—often an important factor in hypertension, especially among blacks—but never eats salt, high blood pressure probably will not develop in that individual. In other words, despite a genetic predisposition to the disease, controllable risk factors, such as diet and exercise, will outweigh the genetic component in most individuals. When both environmental and genetic factors interact to cause illness in a given individual, the disease that results is called a multifactorial disease. Both hypertension and coronary heart disease are multifactorial diseases.

Ethnic origin is another issue directly related to the question of how genetics influences the development of disease in a given individual. Needless to say, you have inherited your racial characteristics—including your level of melanin, the substance that determines the color of your skin—from your parents. Because a larger proportion of blacks than whites suffer from cardiovascular disease, scientists continue to search for a characteristic common to the black race that might explain this phenomenon.

To date, the most important and conclusive link between race and cardiovascular disease involves the way some blacks tend to metabolize salt. As you'll learn in Chapter 2, sodium (a main component of salt) is an integral component of our blood pressure system. It is thought that some people inherit a condition known as "salt-sensitivity," which means that their blood pressure increases (sometimes dramatically) as they consume more salt. Although some whites are salt-sensitive, the tendency is far more common among blacks.

Why would blacks retain salt more than whites? Many scientists, including Dr. Clarence E. Grim of Charles R. Drew University of Medicine and Science in Los Angeles, theorize that many present-day African-Americans may have inherited salt-sensitivity from their African slave ancestors. A large percentage of the slaves destined for America died on the way from Africa because of diarrhea and salt losses, which led to dehydration. Therefore, those who survived were likely to have been those whose bodies could retain more salt and water. In other words, the gene that caused blacks to retain salt was *beneficial* to the race. We descended from those slaves and may have inherited this once beneficial gene; unfortunately, it has become a health hazard by causing blood pressure to rise.

The arguments over genetics and race versus socioeconomic status and lifestyle are only important in a few special areas: if African-Americans metabolize salt differently from whites, for instance, different strategies may be necessary to both prevent and treat hypertension. However, at least at this time, there is little you can do to affect your "uncontrollable risk factors." If you have a family history of hypertension, you run a higher risk of developing the disease than someone who does not. And if you're black, you may be more susceptible to high blood pressure than whites.

Please note, however, that according to several studies, blacks in Africa do not suffer the same high rates of hypertension as black Americans. It is thought that, just as for white Americans, the high-fat, high-salt diets of black Americans, as well as high levels of stress, probably cause most cardiovascular disease.

Controllable Risk Factors

High Blood Cholesterol Experts agree that one of the most important risk factors in the development of cardiovascular disease—especially coronary heart disease—is atherosclerosis, commonly known as hardening of the arteries. Atherosclerosis occurs when the inner layer of the arteries becomes thickened by an accumulation of fats. Cholesterol, a fatty substance that is both consumed in the diet and produced by the body, is a major factor in the development of atherosclerosis. (The role of cholesterol in cardiovascular disease will be discussed in more detail in Chapter 2 and Chapter 6.)

For both blacks and whites alike, the more dietary fat consumed, the more likely the blood vessels and the heart will be damaged. According to the most recent federal surveys, both blacks and whites consume about 35 to 38 percent of their calories as total fat. However, the American Heart Association and other health organizations recommend that no more than 30 percent of our daily total of calories come from fat. In Chapter 6, you'll learn the best way to eliminate this risk factor from your life is by cutting down on the amount of fat you eat every day.

Cigarette Smoking Cigarette smoke is one of the most damaging substances to the human body. Nevertheless, cigarette companies continue to advertise heavily throughout the country, especially in African-American communities. According to statistics collected by the American Heart Association, over 50 million people in the United States still smoke cigarettes on a daily basis. The latest estimates are that more than 430,000 Americans each year die of smoking-related illness.

Smoking has the same devastating effect on the cardiovascular system of both African-Americans and whites. Recent evidence indicates that the proportion of African-American smokers is rising, and fewer blacks are quitting smoking, even as white Americans quit the habit in record numbers. I understand from many of my patients that more of their *children*—particularly their teenaged girls—have started to smoke, even while their parents were attempting to quit.

If you smoke, you are putting yourself at risk for a host of serious health problems. On the other hand, if you quit, you will eliminate one of the most dangerous controllable risk factors for cardiovascular disease. (See Chapter 4 for more information.)

Diabetes Mellitus Diabetes mellitus is defined as an inability to metabolize carbohydrates, specifically sugar. In general, diabetic patients have a much higher incidence of cardiovascular disease, including hypertension and heart disease, than nondiabetics. Experts feel that this is due in part to the fact that diabetics have a much higher level of fat in the bloodstream than nondiabetics. In addition, both the small and the large blood vessels of diabetics tend to thicken abnormally, conditions known as microangiopathy and macroangiopathy. In the famous Framingham Study, a four-decade study in which 5,000 patients from Framingham, Massachusetts, were monitored for cardiovascular disease, 75 percent of the deaths among diabetic men were due to strokes and heart attacks; 80 percent of women diabetics suffered deaths from cardiovascular disease. Although the Framingham Study included few blacks, its results appear to be relevant to the black population as well.

As a group, blacks suffer from diabetes about 33 percent more often than whites. The National Diabetes Data Group reports that black men have a prevalence of diabetes that is 16 percent higher than that of white men and black women have rates more than 50 percent higher than their white counterparts. One reason for the increased incidence of diabetes in the black population is obesity: the Framingham Study showed that patients who were overweight were *eight times more likely to become diabetic* than their thin peers.

Diabetes is listed in this book as a controllable risk factor because it is both preventable in many cases and relatively easy to treat with medication. However, it is a serious condition that requires medical intervention. Table 3 outlines the signs and symptoms of diabetes; should you experience any or all of them, you should see your doctor immediately.

Obesity   Obesity—being more than 20 percent over ideal weight—is a known risk factor for cardiovascular disease for all people, regardless of race, age, or sex. Even ten extra pounds put an incredible burden on the heart and blood vessels; for each pound of excess weight, the heart is forced to pump blood through an additional several hundred extra miles of blood vessels a day. Overweight people also tend to eat too much fat and cholesterol, which contributes to atherosclerosis. Obesity and diabetes are twin threats; most diabetics are overweight, and many overweight individuals will develop diabetes. The combination of hypertension, diabetes, and obesity often leads to heart attack and stroke.

Although an equal proportion of black and white men tend to be overweight, obesity among black women is epidemic. One study showed that 50 percent of African-American women aged twenty-four to fifty-five were obese as compared to 22 percent of white women in the same age group. In one New Haven, Connecticut, survey, the average older black woman was about the same height as the average older white woman, but weighed

TABLE 3 Symptoms of Diabetes

Symptoms usually develop gradually
Frequent urination
Excessive thirst
Sudden weight loss
Weakness and fatigue
Irritability
Nausea and vomiting
Blurred vision or any change in sight
Tingling or numbness in legs, feet, or fingers
Slow healing of cuts (especially the feet)
Frequent skin infections

about 17 pounds more. That black women tend to be heavier than white women may help to explain our greater levels of cardiovascular disease. Why obesity is a such a special problem for black women will be discussed further in Chapter 6.

Sedentary Lifestyle The Surgeon General calls it "Public Enemy Number Two," right behind smoking. Inactivity may be a great way to conserve calories, but that's about all it has going for it. "If we could just get 25 percent of the people who are sedentary up and moving," says Dr. David Satcher, "we could save $4 billion in medical costs."

That's true in part because inactivity is one of the four top risk factors for the development of hypertension, heart attack, and stroke. One of the most obvious reasons for this link is that lack of exercise often leads to obesity since the fewer calories you burn up the more get stored as fat on your body. In addition, vigorous exercise has been linked to lower cholesterol levels.

Along with cigarette smoking and high cholesterol, the lack of exercise is a contributing factor in all types of cardiovascular disease. The Centers for Disease Control and Prevention in Atlanta, Georgia, estimates that upwards of 300,000 deaths per year can be attributed to a sedentary lifestyle. This appears to be equally true in black and white communities; in fact, some studies indicate that blacks may be more sedentary than their white counterparts.

The news is not all grim, however. In fact, the flip side of the startling equation "Inactivity = Disease" is quite encouraging: "Exercise = Disease Prevention." By exercising regularly you can significantly lower your risk of cardiovascular disease.

Salt Intake   Sodium, a main ingredient of salt, is crucial in the regulation of blood pressure; if you consume too much salt and your kidneys are unable to excrete it, the level of fluids in your body will rise. This causes blood pressure to rise, since the vessels and heart must work that much harder to circulate the extra fluid. I once had a patient whose blood pressure was so salt-sensitive that eating a bag of salted potato chips would send her blood pressure out of control.

As discussed above under "Race," exactly why more blacks are salt-sensitive than whites remains unclear. It is true, however, that more than 80 percent of all blacks with hypertension (compared with about 60 percent of white patients) have some degree of salt-sensitivity. Therefore, as you'll learn in Chapter 6, the less table salt and fewer sodium-laden food products you consume, the more you'll reduce your risk of developing hypertension and other cardiovascular diseases.

Alcohol Abuse   Although moderate drinking (two drinks a day or less) has been shown to have no adverse effect on the cardiovascular system, study after study among both black and white populations proves that heavy drinking (more than three drinks per day) significantly raises blood pressure and puts incredible strain on the heart itself. If you have a problem with alcohol, you no doubt realize that there are many medical and personal reasons you should quit. Now you can add the potentially lethal damage you are doing to your heart and blood vessels to the list. For more information about alcohol and your heart, read Chapter 5.

Stress Stress is a buzz word of modern times, one so overused that it has lost much of its meaning. Studying for exams can cause stress, and so can moving, losing a job, getting married, even visiting family members. So what exactly is stress? The Columbia University College of Physicians & Surgeons in *The Complete Home Medical Guide* defines stress as "an imbalance between excessive psychological or physical demands and the ability to cope with them." When your body is faced with these excessive demands, a chain of reactions, known as "the fight-or-flight syndrome," occurs. One of the results of this chain reaction is a marked increase in blood pressure. Usually, the elevated blood pressure returns to normal soon after the stressful situation has been alleviated. However, if an individual is unable to cope with stress on a continuing basis, hypertension and its effects on the heart may result.

Few people would argue that more black Americans live under stress-producing conditions—such as crime-ridden neighborhoods, persistent unemployment, racial discrimination, and poverty—than most whites. Some researchers believe that the anger, frustration, and fear felt by blacks in these conditions have a marked effect on our cardiovascular health.

Perhaps the most important and controversial aspect of the relationship between stress and hypertension among blacks is the effect racism has on our physical selves. We've always known that racism makes us feel angry, bitter, and powerless, but it's only recently that the link between our emotional and physical lives has been confirmed. In one study, twenty-seven black students were shown movies in which racist scenes were depicted. The anger they felt while watching those scenes produced a three-point rise in their blood pressures. Although their pressures returned to normal several moments later, the emotional impact of racism could be directly affecting the health of our cardiovascular system over time.

"If there were no racism in America," claims Dr. Elijah

Saunders, co-author of the book *Hypertension in Blacks* and a cardiologist at the University of Maryland Medical School in Baltimore, "hypertension would be much less of a problem among blacks." Although the dramatic social changes necessary to eliminate racism, crime, and poverty from this society may never be achieved, you as an individual can work to mitigate the effects of stress on your health. Read Chapter 7 for more information.

Taking Control of Your Cardiovascular Health

After reading this chapter and taking the Cardiovascular Self-Test, do you feel you're at risk for high blood pressure and heart disease? If so, you're not alone. Millions of Americans, black and white, have taken up the struggle against the leading cause of death in the modern, industrialized world by changing the kinds of food they eat, the amount of exercise they perform, and by breaking some firmly entrenched bad habits, like smoking and drinking too much.

If you're ready to join them in this endeavor, go on to Chapter 2, where you'll learn the ins and outs of your cardiovascular system. You'll find out how blood is pumped throughout your body, how your heart works as the cardiovascular system center of operation, and what can go wrong if the system is damaged in any way.

IMPORTANT QUESTIONS AND ANSWERS ABOUT CALCULATING YOUR CARDIOVASCULAR RISKS

Q. I was adopted and so don't know about my family's history of high blood pressure or heart disease. How can I judge my risks?

A. If you don't know your family history, concentrate on those factors that you can control. Remember, genetics plays only one role in the development of cardiovascular disease, and there is every reason to believe that dietary and other lifestyle habits are just as important as any family history you may or may not have. Take a look at your adoptive family: Do they eat lots of high-fat foods? Do they exercise on a regular basis? Is the salt shaker an integral part of every meal? If so, you may have inherited some very bad habits from your adoptive family—habits you should try to break as soon as possible.

Q. So far, my blood pressure is normal, but the disease runs in my family. Should I worry about my children's blood pressure?

A. It's never too early to have hypertension, and never too soon to begin a lifelong plan to avoid it. If you have a family history of hypertension or heart disease and have children, it is important to monitor their blood pressure and fat intake carefully. By instilling proper diet and exercise habits in your children from a very young age, you could help prevent them—as well as yourself—from developing cardiovascular disease later in life.

Q. I've been diagnosed with high blood pressure and I also am overweight. Which is more important to control if I want to avoid having a heart attack?

A. Quite frankly, that's a difficult question to answer since both may have an equal impact on your heart. Luckily, however, you may be able to kill two birds with one stone: If you lose weight, your blood pressure is likely to drop at the same time. As stated above, obesity is one of the most important risk factors for hypertension, and hypertension is a leading risk factor for heart disease. If you lose weight and your blood pressure drops, you're that much farther along the road to cardiovascular health.

CHAPTER 2

Understanding Hypertension and Heart Disease

"Ignorance is bliss," so the old saying goes. When it comes to our health, however, there is no doubt that "knowledge is power." But how many of us really understand how our bodies work or how important our cardiovascular systems are to every move we make every day of our lives?

Although more studies have been conducted using white rather than black participants, we know enough to reassure you that, basically speaking, there is no difference between the anatomy of a black man and a white man, or a black woman and a white woman, when it comes to the cardiovascular system. Our hearts and vessels are made of the same muscular material and are located in the same positions as those of whites. Although some parts of our bodies may differ slightly—some scientists believe that blacks tend to have slightly larger kidneys than whites, for example—the similarities far outweigh the differences.

This chapter offers you a primer on the anatomy and physiology of the cardiovascular system so that you can better understand how the general fitness and well-being of every part of your body depends, to a large degree, on the health of your heart and blood vessels.

YOUR CARDIOVASCULAR SYSTEM AT WORK

Your cardiovascular system is made up of a vast network of blood vessels with a hollow muscular pump known as the heart at its center. The heart and blood vessels act as a single system, the purpose of which is to deliver oxygen and nutrients to body organs and to remove waste products from tissue cells. The substance that carries these substances is blood, which is a fluid produced largely in the marrow of bones. Blood is kept in constant circulation by the pumping action of the heart, which sends blood to the lungs to pick up oxygen, and then pumps it to the rest of the body and back to the heart through a system of tubes known as the vascular system (Figure 1).

The vascular system sends blood around the body in a continuous circuit. It is divided into two components: the arteries, which deliver oxygen and nutrients from the heart to the body, and the veins, which return deoxygenated blood back to the heart, where the cycle begins again. Both the arteries and the veins branch off into ever smaller and thinner-walled vessels. The arterioles conduct blood from the arteries to the capillaries, the smallest blood vessels that transmit oxygen and nutrients to the individual body cells and collect waste products. Deoxygenated blood flows first to venules (the smallest veins), which then pass blood along to the veins back to the heart. Stretched end to end, the vessels of your vascular system measure about 60,000 miles, but it takes just one minute for blood to complete one full circuit of the cardiovascular system.

A Healthy Heart

Although the heart weighs less than a pound and is not much larger than the size of a clenched fist, it is the hardest working muscle in your body. Throughout every day of your life, your heart beats approximately once a second and sends about five quarts of blood coursing

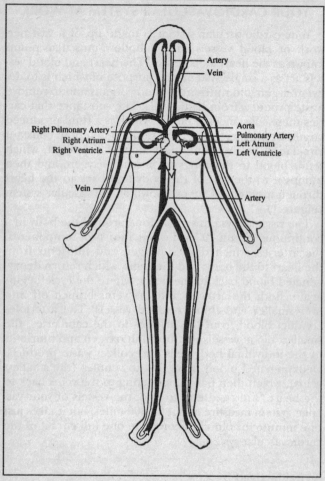

Figure 1 Blood circulates through the body by first entering the right atrium from the veins. To receive oxygen, the blood is pumped from the right atrium into the right ventricle and out through the pulmonary artery to the lungs. Oxygenated blood flows from the lungs into the left side of the heart, from which it is pumped by the left ventricle into the aorta and its branches, called arteries, through the rest of the body.

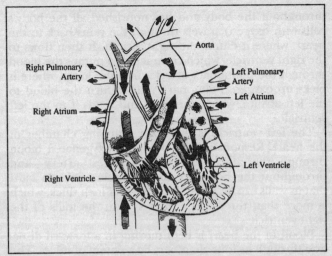

Figure 2 Your heart has four chambers: right and left atria and right and left ventricles. The aorta is the largest artery in the body; it is responsible for pumping oxygenated blood throughout the body. The pulmonary artery takes deoxygenated blood and sends it to the lungs, where blood picks up oxygen.

through your circulatory system every minute. In one year, the average human heart beats 3 million times; the heart of a seventy-year-old has beat more than 2.5 billion times.

Your heart is essentially a sophisticated pump. It is divided into four chambers—the right and left atria and the right and left ventricles (Figure 2). The walls of the chambers are made of a special muscle, the myocardium, that contracts rhythmically under the stimulation of electrical currents. The left and right atria and the left and right ventricles are separated from each other by the septa, a wall of connective tissue and muscle.

Each of the four chambers of the heart serves a particular function in the circulatory system. Oxygen-poor, or deoxygenated blood (blood that has been circulated throughout the body and has nourished all the body's cells with oxygen) travels through the veins back to the heart, where it enters the right atrium. It then flows to the right ventricle, which contracts and pumps the blood through the pulmonary arteries into the lungs, where it picks up oxygen. Pulmonary veins return the blood to the left atrium, which contracts and sends it to the left ventricle.

The left ventricle is the main pumping chamber of the heart. Responsible for pumping oxygenated blood through the aorta—the body's largest artery—and throughout the body, the left ventricle works so hard that its walls can be more than one-half inch thick, which is more than three times thicker than the walls of the right ventricle.

Blood in the heart is kept moving in a forward direction through its four chambers by a system of valves. The valves open to let blood through when the chambers contract and then quickly shut tight to prevent blood from flowing backward as the chambers relax. In fact, the familiar "lub-dub" sound of the heartbeat is created by the snapping shut of the valves and from the turbulence produced by the flow of blood.

Like any other organ or tissue in the body, the heart muscle is fed by oxygen and nutrients in the blood. The heart supplies blood to itself through two coronary arteries, the right and the left. The coronary arteries stem from the aorta and run around the outside of the heart. After giving off its oxygen in the heart, the blood travels through the coronary veins and drains directly into the right atrium, where it joins the deoxygenated blood coming into the heart from the rest of the body.

Later in this chapter, you'll learn what can happen to this remarkable organ if it does not receive the blood it needs from the coronary arteries. In the meantime, let's see how blood manages to make its way around the body.

Healthy Blood Pressure

You hear about blood pressure often enough; you remember your grandmother telling you that all your misbehaving was "gonna get her pressure up," and you knew that was something to avoid, for your own good as well as your grandmother's health. Your doctor takes your blood pressure whenever you go in for a visit; a community center sponsors Saturday morning blood pressure checks in your neighborhood. But you still wonder what exactly blood pressure is. What are they really measuring when they take your blood pressure reading and what does that reading mean?

In studying how our cardiovascular system works, we must examine many different organ systems in addition to the circulatory system: the hormones our body produces, the ways in which our kidneys function, and how the nervous system coordinates our bodily functions all affect how hard and how often our heart beats, and the rate at which the blood flows through our vascular system.

With each heartbeat, about two to three ounces of freshly oxygenated blood are forced out of the heart and into general circulation. To keep the blood flowing through the 60,000 miles of vessels, a certain amount of force is required. This force is called *blood pressure*. At the head of the blood pressure system is the heart, but the arterioles also play a large role in determining the amount of pressure in the vessels throughout the body. To raise blood pressure, the arterioles narrow; to lower it, they open up.

While the force required to keep blood moving through the body originates in the heart and vessels, three other body systems—kidneys, the nervous system, and the endocrine system (which produces hormones)—work together to control the blood pressure.

The Kidneys and Blood Pressure   Blood pressure is affected by the level of fluid circulating in the body and it is the kidneys, a pair of bean-shaped organs located at the base of the abdominal cavity, that regulate this fluid level by either retaining salt and water or by eliminating salt and water through the urine. As the level of fluid in the body increases, the heart and the vessels are forced to work harder simply to move the excess fluid through the body. In addition, when there is too much fluid in body tissue, the tissue becomes stiff, making it difficult for blood to enter and nourish the cells. Because the arteries must contract harder to push the blood out into the tissues, the blood pressure goes up.

The Nervous System and Blood Pressure The part of the nervous system that controls unconscious functions such as blood pressure and respiration—called the autonomic nervous system—is responsible for sending messages to and from the heart, arteries, and kidneys. A collection of nerve cells, called vasomotor nerves and located in arterial muscle tissue, for instance, regulate the expansion and contraction of the vessel walls. When body cells require more oxygen or nutrients, the vasomotor nerves assist in accommodating these changes. When we exercise, for instance, our voluntary muscles need more oxygen; our arteries will expand to bring more blood into the area.

Other groups of sympathetic nerve cells, called baroreceptors, also help to control the body's blood pressure. Baroreceptors assist in maintaining the blood pressure at a relatively constant state by stimulating reflex mechanisms in the brain that allow the body to adapt to changes in blood pressure by dilating or constricting the blood vessels.

Your Hormones at Work Working to deliver the nervous system messages to the heart and blood vessels are a group of chemicals called hormones, which are produced by the endocrine system. Hormones produced by the adrenal gland, an endocrine gland located on top of the kidney, play a particularly important role in controlling blood pressure. When the sympathetic nervous system senses danger or stress, for instance, it signals the adrenal gland to release its two primary hormones, epinephrine and norepinephrine, also known as the "fight-or-flight" stress hormones. Both epinephrine and norepinephrine make the heart beat faster and cause the blood vessels to constrict, which raises blood pressure.

Aldosterone is another hormone important to the regulation of blood pressure. Aldosterone works within the kidneys to regulate the amount of water and salt in the body. When aldosterone is secreted by the adrenal gland, located on the top of the kidney, more salt and water is retained; as discussed above, when fluid levels rise in the body, so too does blood pressure.

Another hormone released by the kidney is called renin. Renin works in combination with another hormone, angiotensin. Whenever the kidney senses the need to raise the blood pressure, it secretes renin into the bloodstream, setting off a chain of events that ends with angiotensin being converted to another hormone, angiotensin II, which then causes the walls of the arteries to constrict, which raises the blood pressure. Angiotensin II also stimulates the release of aldosterone, which, you'll remember, causes the kidneys to retain salt and water. The renin-angiotensin-aldosterone system is not completely understood as yet, but research has shown that it is indeed a crucial factor in the development of high blood pressure.

What Causes Hypertension?

Exactly what causes high blood pressure is as yet poorly understood in most cases. In fact, 90 to 95 percent of all cases of hypertension are classified as *essential* hypertension in which no precise cause for it can be identified. Because the nature of the blood pressure system is so complicated and involves so many different components, it is difficult to pinpoint exactly what causes high blood pressure in a given individual. As we've seen, the vascular, hormonal, renal, and autonomic nervous systems are all involved, working in complex unity to regulate blood flow throughout the body. Often, a patient at risk of developing hypertension may have more than one abnormality in more than one of those systems.

In about 10 percent of cases of hypertension, an underlying, or *secondary*, cause of the disease process exists. Secondary hypertension is caused by another condition, like kidney disease or hyperthyroidism, or it may be due to an external factor, such as drug abuse or treatment with certain prescription drugs. Use of cocaine, for instance, is known to elevate blood pressure, as is long-term alcohol abuse. The birth control pill, which consists of the female hormones progesterone and estrogen, may cause some women to retain water, which increases blood volume and leads to added pressure in the blood vessels. When drug and alcohol abuse stops, or when a woman ceases to take the pill, blood pressure often returns to normal or is more easily managed in a very short time.

In the case of secondary hypertension, once the underlying cause is identified and corrected, the blood pressure usually returns to normal. One such case was that of a twenty-eight-year-old black woman who was referred to me because of poorly controlled hypertension. Her young age made me suspicious of a secondary cause of her high blood pressure. After an extensive exam and several tests, I found that she was suffering from a severe narrowing of one of the arteries that supplies blood to the left kidney. Once this problem was corrected, her hypertension was almost completely resolved.

Essential hypertension, however, is especially frustrating because it has no known cause and therefore no cure. Fortunately, however, hypertension is usually relatively easy to control through lifestyle changes and medication. In Chapter 3, you'll learn how high blood pressure is measured and how hypertension is diagnosed and evaluated by your physician.

DOWN THE ROAD: THE LONG-TERM EFFECTS OF HYPERTENSION

Perhaps you're thinking, "I feel perfectly fine, so I don't need to worry about my blood pressure." If so, you could be endangering your health. While those with severe hypertension may be symptomatic, people with mild and moderate cases usually feel pretty good. If you wait until you feel sick, your high blood pressure may have already caused damage to the brain, kidneys, eyes, and of course, the heart. In combination with other factors, such as cigarette smoking, diabetes, hardening of the arteries (atherosclerosis), and obesity, high blood pressure is the leading killer of Americans through heart disease, stroke, and kidney disease.

The Brain

Stroke is the third most frequent cause of death in the United States among the population as a whole as well as among blacks. Hypertension is an extremely significant contributor to the likelihood of stroke: it is estimated that strict control of high blood pressure could prevent over one half of strokes in blacks.

Strokes occur in a number of different ways: Atherosclerosis (the blockage of blood vessels by fatty plaques) is responsible for a majority of strokes. Aneurisms (the ballooning out of vessels) may result in strokes when the affected blood vessels rupture because they are weakened over time by high blood pressure. Blood clots stop the blood flow to the brain in another common type of cerebrovascular event. Any of these incidents cuts off blood flow to the brain, resulting in the death of brain tissue. Stroke then is both a neurological disease and a cardiovascular disease because it is caused by damage to the blood vessels that feed the brain. In more than 150,000 cases every year, stroke results in death.

In addition to full-blown strokes, another type of vascular disease that affects the brain is called a transient ischemic attack, or TIA. A TIA occurs when the blood supply to a part of the brain is temporarily stopped, due to a blood clot or to an artery that has been closed off because of atherosclerosis. The part of the brain this vessel feeds then does not receive the blood it needs to function properly. Although the event usually lasts only a few moments until the vessel clears itself of its obstruction or another nearby vessel assists in bringing blood to that part of the brain, a TIA is often called a "mini-stroke" and is a warning to the patient that he or she is suffering from cardiovascular disease.

Even when strokes aren't fatal, they are often debilitating; in fact, stroke is the leading cause of disability among older adults in the United States today. Strokes can cause paralysis, speech loss, hearing loss, blindness, memory loss, and can have many other devastating results. A tragic example of a stroke's effects involves my close friend's mother, a black woman in her late forties who had severe high blood pressure. For some unknown reason, she stopped taking her antihypertensive medication. One day, my friend called me in a state of panic. His mother had been hospitalized with a severe stroke. He wanted to know what he could do. Unfortunately, the damage done by the stroke was so extensive that she was never able to fully recover and my friend decided to put her in a nursing home so that her many medical needs could be met.

I hope this information has frightened you a bit so that you'll take more control over your health. The fact is, most strokes are preventable *if you control your high blood pressure*. One extensive study, the Hypertensive Detection and Follow-Up Program (HDFP) looked into the effects of various levels of treatment of hypertension on stroke prevention. The participants in the study were divided randomly into two groups. One group continued to see their personal doctor or visit their regular clinic, with no particularly aggressive efforts to keep their blood pressure down. The other group went to special HDFP clinics that required patients to maintain very strict control over their blood pressure.

The study participants were followed for five years, and the results were pretty dramatic. In black participants, there was a 22.4 percent lower death rate among those in the second group, and there was a 10 percent lower death rate among whites in the second group. So, while both whites and blacks benefited from strict control of blood pressure, blacks benefited far more. The results for stroke incidence were even more astounding: There was a 45.3 percent greater reduction in the incidence of stroke in the second group, with black women having the greatest reduction—45.5 percent. Even patients with mild hypertension had 45 percent fewer strokes as a result of strict hypertension control.

The Kidneys

Longstanding uncontrolled hypertension is probably the most common cause of partial and/or complete kidney failure among blacks. Hypertension can cause the renal blood vessels to thicken and harden, making it extremely difficult to nourish the kidneys with oxygen. Without oxygen, the kidney cannot remove all of the toxins from the blood, a condition known as kidney failure. Kidney failure produces a variety of symptoms, including nausea, weakness, and fatigue, among others.

Often the patient with renal failure will require kidney dialysis. In effect, kidney dialysis provides the patient suffering from acute or chronic renal failure with a way to excrete the wastes from the blood without using his or her own kidneys. There are several methods of kidney dialysis, including hemodialysis, which filters the blood through a purifying machine and then returns it to the body. Another method, peritoneal dialysis, uses the patient's own peritoneum—lining of the abdominal cavity—as a dialysis membrane. A solution of glucose (a form of sugar) and mineral salts is periodically injected into and withdrawn from the cavity. When the fluid comes into contact with the blood vessels in the peritoneum, it forces waste products from the vessels into the fluid in the peritoneum. The fluid is then removed from the body. Another method, called continuous ambulatory peritoneal dialysis, uses the same method, but uses a surgically implanted tube that allows the patient to remove the fluid him- or herself at home.

I have seen any number of patients who have suffered complete or partial loss of kidney function as a result of untreated hypertension. One particularly heartbreaking case was that of a twenty-six-year-old black man who had been suffering from headaches he'd been trying to ignore. One night he had an extremely severe headache he just couldn't shake. When he came to the hospital, his blood pressure was 240/120. He told me he'd been having trouble urinating and that there was often blood in his urine. Blood tests confirmed that he had severe renal failure due to longstanding uncontrolled hypertension—not something he expected at twenty-six—and that he'd have to be on dialysis (or have a kidney transplant) for the rest of his life.

As with many other complications from hypertension, blacks have a greater risk of developing end stage renal disease (ESRD) than other ethnic groups, and hypertension as a cause of ESRD is seen more often in blacks than in nonblacks. In one five-year Baltimore study, 50 percent of blacks, as opposed to 18 percent of whites, had hypertension as the listed cause of ESRD.

The Eyes

Over time, hypertension can cause serious damage to the small, delicate blood vessels of the eyes. Retinal hemorrhage, or bleeding due to ruptured arteries or veins in the retina and detached retinas (the separation of the blood vessels from the retina) are the most dreaded eye problems caused by hypertension. Both conditions can result in blindness. A former patient once came to me complaining that his vision was getting progressively worse. A physical exam revealed that his blood pressure was extremely high and his hypertension had been uncontrolled for some time. As a result, blood vessels in his eyes had ruptured, causing swelling in the part of the eye—called the macula lutea—responsible for accurate vision. Once we were able to bring his blood pressure down to a normal level and with careful follow-up and care, this patient's eyesight returned to normal.

The Heart

Uncontrolled hypertension can damage the heart in many different ways. In the next section of this chapter, you'll learn about coronary heart disease and how hypertension contributes to its development. Hypertension also directly causes a condition known as left ventricular hypertrophy (LVH), or an increase in the thickness of the left ventricular wall. This is a potentially serious complication of hypertension.

When you have high blood pressure, your heart has to work harder to pump blood. Since your heart is a muscle, the more work it has to do, the larger it gets—just as your biceps get larger when you lift weights. The left ventricle, as you will remember, pumps oxygenated blood to the tissues. It therefore has the most work to do to begin with, and when the added stress of hypertension complicates matters further, the left ventricle becomes extremely overworked. The left ventricular wall, which is now contracting with more force each time it has to pump blood, becomes thicker over time.

LVH causes many cardiac complications. As the wall thickens, it becomes more difficult for the ventricle to expand and hence to completely fill up with blood. Blood may back up into the blood vessels in the lungs, putting more pressure on these vessels and causing shortness of breath. If this process continues and the pressure gets very high, *pulmonary edema,* a flooding of the lungs with fluid, can result. Pulmonary edema, which causes a severe shortness of breath, is a medical emergency and is potentially fatal if not treated immediately.

LVH can also cause *angina*—recurring sharp pains or tightness in the chest. The thickened muscle of the left ventricle can essentially squeeze the small blood vessels, called arterioles and capillaries, until they have been obliterated. The tissue nourished by these vessels is deprived of oxygen for a short period of time, and the pain of angina is the result.

If your hypertension remains uncontrolled, LVH will progress to a thinning of the heart muscle (because of tissue death as noted above). The heart then gets larger, or dilated, and loses much of its pumping power. This results in congestive heart failure (the heart can no longer pump enough to circulate the blood throughout the body) and, potentially, end stage heart disease. LVH is also a risk factor for developing coronary artery disease.

There do seem to be some drugs that can reduce the thickness of the left ventricle, but their degrees of effectiveness vary widely. Some of these treatments have been shown to reduce LVH in as little as six weeks. However, this is no proof that such early regression of LVH will remain after longer periods of treatment. Perhaps most frustrating is the fact that though it is clear that increased left ventricular mass contributes to increased cardiovascular risk, there is no evidence that regression of LVH reduces that risk. In other words, if hypertension has caused LVH, there is no guarantee that your risk of developing serious heart problems will be reduced even if the left ventricular wall returns to normal size.

The only sure way to reduce the risk of LVH and further cardiovascular complications from hypertension is to keep your blood pressure under control in the first place. In Chapter 3, you'll learn more about how hypertension is diagnosed and, in Chapter Seven, how it is treated with drugs. In the meantime, it's important to learn about another related and quite serious threat to your cardiovascular system.

CORONARY HEART DISEASE

Coronary heart disease is a variety of disorders of the heart muscle (myocardium) that result in restriction or blockage of its blood supply. The disorders range from the warning pain called angina to the injury and even death of parts of the heart muscle caused by a heart attack.

Almost all cases of coronary heart disease are due to the progressive narrowing of the coronary arteries, which supply heart tissue with the blood it needs to survive. The narrowing is caused by atherosclerosis, a disease in which plaques made of fatty substances and blood clots collect on the inner wall of one or both coronary arteries. The buildup of atherosclerotic plaque is usually a gradual process, one that may take decades before any symptoms of cardiovascular damage appear. However, there are some diseases, such as familial hypercholesterolemia, in which atherosclerosis accelerates quite rapidly and at a remarkably early age—even in childhood. Hypertension, too, may accelerate the process greatly in individuals who do not control their high blood pressure.

Hypertension accelerates the process of atherosclerosis by creating areas of injured tissue along arterial walls that are more prone to collect deposits of fat and cholesterol. When blood pressure is high, blood pushes against the arterial walls with greater than normal force and thus damages the lining of the arteries. As a result of this injury, specialized blood cells responsible for healing attach to the damaged places, creating plaques that can block the flow of blood. Over time, lipids (or fats) accumulate at the site of the damage, further blocking the artery.

In Chapter 3, you'll learn how blood lipid levels are measured and what the results of such a test may mean to the health of your cardiovascular system. In the meantime, it is important to understand how atherosclerotic disease can damage your heart.

TABLE 4 Symptoms of a Heart Attack

Nausea
Excessive sweating
Crushing pain in the chest or arm
Dizziness
Fatigue
Breathlessness

Angina: The Heart's Warning System

Ischemic heart disease occurs when the blood supply to the heart is reduced as a result of atherosclerosis of the coronary arteries or when the heart goes into spasm. ("Ischemia" means lack of adequate blood supply.) In some cases, such narrowing can occur without producing any discomfort, a condition referred to as "silent ischemia."

However, many patients experience pain called angina pectoris as their heart muscle becomes deprived of oxygen. Angina usually occurs when the heart's workload increases and it cannot get enough oxygen to enable it to perform, such as during or after exercise or some other strenuous physical activity or when a person is experiencing strong emotion (like anger).

The pain of angina is usually located in the center of the chest, but may radiate to or occur only in the neck, shoulder, arm, or lower jaw. No permanent damage to the heart occurs during an angina attack, but it is a warning sign that your cardiovascular system is in trouble. You should see a doctor as soon as possible because of the danger that narrowing of your arteries will continue or that the plaque will rupture suddenly, causing a heart attack.

Heart Attack

In the fall of 1990, one of my patients, a fifty-six-year-old black man, complained of chest pain one night right after dinner. Thinking it was a simple case of indigestion,

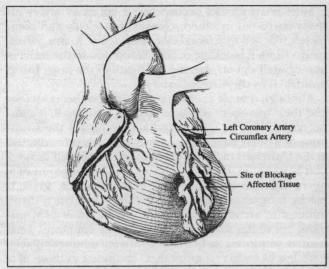

Figure 3 Myocardial ischemia (lack of sufficient oxygen to the heart) often causes angina pectoris—pain that may radiate from the center of the chest up to the arms, neck, and jaw.

he managed to ignore it for more than twelve hours. When the pain finally grew too great and he realized it wasn't going to go away, he got himself to the emergency room. Within moments he found out that he was having a severe heart attack. If he had recognized his symptoms as those of a heart attack and come to the hospital sooner, we could have prevented some of the damage that was done to his heart.

Heart attack is the most serious form of ischemic heart disease. A heart attack occurs when an area of the heart muscle is so severely deprived of blood that it can no longer survive. A heart attack is also called a *myocardial infarction: Myo* means muscle, *cardio* relates to the heart, and *infarct* is a word used to describe the area of dead tissue (Figure 3).

Most heart attacks occur when a coronary artery already narrowed by atherosclerosis is suddenly and completely blocked by a blood clot or muscular spasm. When such a sudden blockage occurs, blood flow to the heart is immediately cut off, causing the death of the heart tissue nourished by the affected artery.

Although a more thorough discussion of heart attacks and their treatment will take place in Chapter 9, it's important for you to understand and recognize the symptoms of a heart attack now (Table 4). A study conducted at the University of North Carolina at Chapel Hill showed that blacks are less likely to recognize the symptoms of a heart attack or to receive medical treatment. In fact, blacks took about twenty-three hours and thirty-three minutes to arrive at a hospital after the onset of symptoms, but whites suffering from the same symptoms were treated within eight hours and fifteen minutes. Blacks were less likely to recognize their symptoms as those of a heart attack, instead attributing them to heartburn, indigestion, or simply being out of breath. Studies show that patients who receive treatment within six hours of the onset of symptoms have the best chances of making a full recovery.

Currently, nine out of every ten heart attack victims who reach the hospital survive the attack. Recovery from a heart attack depends on the size of the infarct, coexisting complications like heart failure, and the patient's general health. In some cases, a heart attack may be so mild as to go unnoticed: believe it or not, a large number of people who have severe or fatal heart attacks have previously had minor heart attacks of which they were totally unaware.

For many reasons discussed earlier in this chapter, many African-Americans choose not to visit doctors, especially for an illness that produces few or no symptoms. However, if after reading these two chapters, you feel you're at risk of hypertension or coronary heart disease, it is essential that you visit your doctor. In the next chapter, you'll find out how hypertension and heart disease are diagnosed, what to expect from your physician, and how to establish a mutually beneficial relationship with your physician.

IMPORTANT QUESTIONS AND ANSWERS ABOUT UNDERSTANDING HYPERTENSION AND CORONARY HEART DISEASE

Q. I have frequent headaches that are sometimes so painful that I get dizzy and feel nauseous. Am I suffering from hypertension? Could it be a warning sign of a heart attack or stroke?

A. Maybe. But your symptoms also resemble those associated with a number of other conditions. See your physician immediately, especially if you have any reason to believe you may have hypertension because of a family history or other risk factors. The only way to know for sure whether or not you have high blood pressure is to have a thorough physical exam.

Q. I'm a forty-year-old woman who suffers from chest pain my doctor calls angina. Does angina mean that I'm having a heart attack?

A. Absolutely not. Not all pain related to the heart means that there is death of heart tissue, which is the real definition of a heart attack. However, angina does mean that the heart muscle is not getting enough blood and oxygen to do its work and is thus at increased risk of having a heart attack. Since the heart is receiving *some* blood, however, no tissue death results. If your angina is caused by atherosclerosis or hypertension, you should attempt to eliminate as many risk factors as possible in order to reverse the disease process before a heart attack does occur.

Q. Is a heart attack always fatal?

A. Around two-thirds of the estimated 1.1 million Americans who have a heart attack in any given year survive the event. But at least 250,000 people a year die suddenly within one hour of experiencing the symptoms of a heart attack and before they can reach a hospital. It is in this group of patients that blacks are represented in a disproportionate number, mainly because we tend not to recognize the symptoms of a heart attack or to get to a hospital quickly enough to avoid major damage to the organ.

Q. I have hypertension, and my doctor told me I'd probably have it for the rest of my life. Does that mean that I'll have a heart attack or stroke or kidney disease?

A. Only if you fail to *control* your hypertension. If you do not follow your doctor's prescribed method of treatment, which may involve drug therapy (see Chapter 8 for more information), dietary and/or exercise measures, you may indeed develop serious health problems because of your high blood pressure. However, *controlled* hypertension, although requiring constant monitoring, should not cause you to feel or become ill.

CHAPTER 3

Establishing a Medical Diagnosis

Harlan D.*, a black man of about forty-five years, came to my office one day complaining of fatigue, headaches, and episodes of dizziness. When I asked him how long he'd been feeling poorly, he admitted that it had been so long since he'd felt really well, he couldn't tell me exactly when the first symptoms had occurred—it may well have been years. When asked what took him so long to come to me for a checkup, Harlan told me that he didn't think his minor complaints were worth a visit to the doctor. After all, he'd managed to get himself to work and do his job as a construction worker every day, so why bother a doctor?

As stated more than once in this text, hypertension and heart disease are often silent killers: you may not be aware that you are ill before significant damage has been done. Although visiting your doctor when you don't feel sick may seem silly, it is the only way to head off the serious consequences of hypertension and heart disease. You may think you don't have the time or money to go to a doctor, but the truth is that if you wait until you are

---

*All names of patients have been changed to protect their privacy.

sick, you will spend far more time and money at your doctor's office and the hospital than you would if you nipped your health problems in the bud.

Luckily, Harlan caught his problem in time. He was indeed suffering from serious high blood pressure, which had already begun to damage the vessels in his eyes and probably had helped accelerate the buildup of plaque in one of his coronary arteries. If he had waited much longer, he might have permanently lost his sight, suffered a major heart attack, or both.

As discussed in the Introduction, lack of health insurance and the scarcity of medical facilities explain some of the resistance to medical care among many sectors of the black community. In fact, a study performed by the National Institutes of Health and published in the journal, *Diabetes/Metabolism,* pointed out that white Americans have approximately 40 percent more visits to office-based physicians every year than blacks. In addition, blacks tend to fear and distrust the mostly white medical establishment, perhaps because our health care priorities have been ignored for so long.

Cultural reasons for this disparity may also apply: I had one elderly patient, Mavis B., for instance, who waited to come to me until her legs were so swollen and stiff—a clear sign of heart failure—that she could barely walk. But before I could begin to examine her, she asked if I was a "root doctor." When I told her no, Mavis left, without allowing me to explain that I understood her beliefs and that we would work together every step of the way. This poor, suffering woman might have been helped, but probably because her concerns and beliefs had been dismissed out of hand by other physicians—mostly white physicians—she felt she couldn't trust me either. Such a mistrust of modern medicine, however well founded in our culture and history, may be killing us.

No matter what your reason for avoiding your doctor, if you feel you're at risk for cardiovascular disease, make an appointment for a checkup today. It may save your life.

DIAGNOSING CARDIOVASCULAR DISEASE

There are several tests that your doctor might perform to determine whether or not you suffer from cardiovascular disease. The first thing your doctor will do is take a complete medical history. When taking a history, your doctor is most concerned with your own past medical history, as well as any medication you are on. He or she will want to know whether you or any other members of your family have been diagnosed with hypertension, heart disease, kidney disease, diabetes, or have experienced symptoms of stroke.

It will prove a great help if you think about the kinds of information your doctor will need before you go in. Completing "Your Cardiovascular Self-Test" in Chapter 1 will help you give your doctor more complete and accurate answers. If your parents and/or grandparents are no longer living, ask aunts, uncles, or cousins if they remember your parents or grandparents taking any medications, or if they remember what they died of. One of the most positive aspects of many black families is their physical and emotional closeness: cousins, uncles, and aunts are likely to live next door or in the next town, and therefore, it is easy to ask them about the medical history of someone on their side of the family who has passed away. Of course, the best way to learn the medical histories of your family members is to ask them while you still can. If they seem reluctant to tell you, assure them that you are not trying to get in their business, but you need to know to protect your own health.

The last part of your medical history exam will focus on lifestyle factors. Your doctor will ask if you smoke, and if so, how many cigarettes you smoke each day. He or she will want to know if you drink alcohol and how often, what kinds of foods you eat, how much salt you use, whether you exercise and how often, your level of stress, and if you use any drugs, especially cocaine. You should also tell your doctor if you take any over-the-counter (nonprescription) drugs regularly. These include cold remedies (particularly decongestants) and diet pills.

Be honest. This is not a morality test. If your doctor seems to disapprove of some of your habits, it is not because he or she thinks you've broken some ethical code or because he or she thinks you're a bad or weak person (and if it is, you should look for a new doctor). Instead, the information will help your doctor more accurately and efficiently assess your health. If you embellish the truth, or hide it, you're only hurting yourself. All information taken in a medical history and all medical records and test results are strictly confidential. They can't be released to your employer or anyone else without your permission. Remember, in order for your relationship with your physician to be helpful, you must be honest and thorough about your body.

In the physical exam, your doctor is looking for several things. He or she first wants to verify your blood pressure. Second, he or she wants to make sure there is nothing to suggest secondary hypertension—an underlying cause such as kidney disease—which could be causing your blood pressure to become elevated. Finally, he or she must be certain that hypertension and/or atherosclerosis has not damaged any of your organs, including your heart.

The order in which your doctor decides to perform the physical exam is arbitrary, but for simplicity's sake, we'll start from the head and work our way down. Your doctor will first look into your eyes with an instrument called an ophthalmoscope, which shines a very bright light onto your retina. The blood vessels here are easily visible, and your doctor will be able to tell if hypertension and/or atherosclerosis has damaged them. He or she will probably feel your neck for an enlarged thyroid gland, since an overactive thyroid gland can occasionally cause hypertension, and he or she will check the carotid arteries in the neck. He or she will palpate the abdomen, checking for abnormalities in the kidneys, and will take the pulses in your arms and legs. In this way, your doctor will be able to assess the condition of your blood vessels throughout your body. In addition, your doctor will carefully examine your heart and measure your blood pressure as part of your general physical examination.

MEASURING BLOOD PRESSURE

An important part of the exam involves taking the blood pressure. A blood pressure measurement focuses on the two stages of heart action, as you may remember from Chapter 2: (1) systole, during which the heart pumps blood out to the arteries, and (2) diastole, during which the heart is at rest and filling with blood. Blood pressure is at its highest point during systole and its lowest during diastole.

Blood pressure is measured by an instrument called a sphygmomanometer, which allows physicians to calculate how hard the heart is pumping and how much the blood vessels must contract to push the blood along. The sphygmomanometer is made up of three components: an inflatable rubber cuff attached to a gauge filled with mercury that resembles a thermometer and a stethoscope. As air is pumped into the cuff, the level of mercury is raised within the gauge's column, which is delineated in measurements of milliliters.

To take your blood pressure, your doctor will first snugly wrap the cuff around your upper arm and then pump air into it until the cuff is tight enough to keep blood from flowing. He or she then places the stethoscope on the arm just below the elbow. Listening carefully, the physician slowly releases air from the cuff and waits to hear the sound of the first spurt of blood as it passes through the artery; this represents the systolic pressure, the maximum pressure that is generated to push the blood from the heart and move it through the arteries. When your doctor hears that spurt of blood, he or she will note the position of the mercury in the column; that is the first number of the blood pressure reading.

The doctor then allows more and more air out of the cuff. At the point when the cuff is no longer restricting the blood flow and the doctor hears no sound at all, the diastolic pressure is read. This is the pressure that the arteries exert on the blood while the heart is filling up; it is the pressure in the circulation between heartbeats.

If your blood pressure is, say, 120/80, it means that your doctor heard the first spurt of blood flow through your artery when the pressure in the cuff pushed the mercury up to 120 millimeters on the gauge and the mercury had fallen to 80 millimeters by the time all external pressure had been removed. Your doctor will then measure the blood pressure in your other arm and compare the two results. If the blood pressure is high in one arm and low in the other, it may indicate that high blood pressure and/or atherosclerosis has already caused significant blockage in the vessels; since less blood is reaching one arm, the blood pressure in that arm will be lower. In this case, further tests may be required.

Although a blood pressure exam is relatively simple and completely painless, it's important to realize that it's not always 100 percent accurate.

One of the most common causes of an inaccurate reading involves defects in the sphygmomanometer itself. Often the cuff—the part of the device that wraps around your upper arm—doesn't fit properly. If you find that the cuff fails to encircle at least two-thirds of your arm from the elbow to the shoulder, ask your doctor for a different size. If the cuff is too big, a child-sized one may fit a bit better. For those of you with particularly large upper arms—a special problem for many obese black women—a cuff usually used to measure blood pressure from the thighs may better suit your needs.

Your own physical condition at the time of the exam is another important factor in obtaining an accurate reading. Any number of things could cause your blood pressure to rise for a short period of time, giving you a high blood pressure reading when, in fact, your blood pressure is normal most of the time. Running to make your appointment on time or smoking two or three cigarettes in the waiting room, for instance, will cause your blood pressure to appear to be quite high, although moments later it will usually return to a normal level.

Your emotional state also has an impact on your blood pressure reading. Are you terrified of going to the doctor? Some people are, especially those who are unaccustomed to going to a physician, and when they have a blood pressure reading taken in the doctor's office, it is often within the hypertensive range. This is known as "The White Coat Syndrome," and it may be more common among black than white patients because blacks tend to fear and mistrust the medical establishment. In fact, this syndrome could be termed "The White *Man* in the White Coat Syndrome" for black Americans.

Any number of my own patients have high blood pressures on their first visits to the clinic. Once they feel more comfortable with me, however, I notice that their blood pressure readings are normal. One young woman, Shaundra C., was very timid and reserved, and a little fidgety; when I took her blood pressure, it was quite high. After a few minutes of chatting and joking with me, Shaundra was able to see me not as some threatening doctor, but as someone she could really relate to. She eventually got more comfortable, and when her blood pressure was taken again, it was completely normal.

For all of these reasons, the Joint National Committee on Detection, Evaluation and Treatment of High Blood Pressure recommends that more than one and preferably three separate blood pressure readings be taken during a physical exam and an average reading calculated. If you have an averaged reading that's particularly high, your doctor will probably recommend that you come back in a few days or a week to take another reading. If it is normal on that occasion, he or she may want to give you yet another set of readings a week or two after that. The average of these three averaged readings should give you an accurate measure of your blood pressure.

How high is too high? Although general categories have been established, the truth is that no exact dividing line exists between normal and high blood pressure. Blood pressure readings fall into five separate categories that are applicable to black and white Americans alike. Anything reading between 110/70 and 140/90 is within the *normal range*. However, someone with normal blood pressure who has a family history of hypertension and/or is overweight, salt-sensitive, or sedentary may not stay within the normal range for very long.

Stage 1 hypertension is any reading of 140 to 159 systolic and 90 to 99 diastolic. Most of the estimated 60 million people with high blood pressure in the United States fall into this category. Like those with normal pressure but at high risk, most stage I hypertensives can treat their disease with diet, salt restriction, and weight control.

A reading of 160 to 179 systolic and 100 to 109 diastolic indicates *stage 2 hypertension*. The heart, vessels, and kidney are at greater risk of damage. Depending on the general health of the individual, changes in diet and exercise habits may be enough to bring blood pressure back into the normal range.

Any reading of 180 to 209 systolic and 110 to 199 diastolic is considered *stage 3 hypertension*. Both *stage 3* and *stage 4 hypertension* (which is any reading above 210/120) are serious conditions requiring medical attention.

Although these categories give you a general idea how to evaluate blood pressure readings, judging your own personal reading is another matter. Let's say, as we did at the beginning of this section, that you were given a clean bill of blood pressure health with a reading of 135/85. Doesn't that mean that your heart and vessels are not being damaged?

That's a difficult question to answer with any certainty. Blood pressure, as we've seen, is a relative matter. A very few people with blood pressures well above the normal range never show signs of cardiovascular disease. Most studies, however, have shown that the higher the blood pressure, the greater the risks of disease—*even if they fall within the normal range.* Generally speaking, someone with a blood pressure of 110/70 runs fewer cardiovascular health risks than someone with a blood pressure of 120/80. In turn, the person with a 120/80 reading may fare better in the long run than the person whose pressure is measured at 135/85.

For most people, then, the lower the blood pressure the better. Your own "perfect" blood pressure is determined by your weight, height, age, and other individual physical characteristic factors.

The Cardiac Exam

Your doctor will listen to your heart to check its size, rate at which it beats, and the types of sounds it makes. The standard stethoscope he or she will use consists of a Y-shaped plastic tube with an earpiece at each end. The stethoscope is equipped with a diaphragm that picks up and magnifies sounds when pressed against the chest wall.

Often, your doctor will perform a test called an *electrocardiogram.* This test gives a record of the heart's electrical patterns while at rest. In a healthy person, the passage of electrical impulses through the heart follows a regular sequence. If there is any abnormality, this pattern is altered. By observing the patterns your heart produces, your doctor can identify areas of the heart muscle that may have been damaged by coronary heart disease, as well as detect thickening of heart muscle walls or irregular heartbeats (arrhythmias).

The electrocardiogram is performed by attaching electrodes to the chest, wrists, and ankles. In most cases, an EKG is performed while you are lying down. Although usually completely painless, some patients complain that the substance used to attach the electrodes causes temporary skin irritation.

Your doctor may also decide to give you a *stress test* to check the electrical patterns of the heart during exertion. Usually, you will be asked to walk or jog on a treadmill or ride a stationary bike for this test, and your heart will be monitored continuously by an EKG. The idea is to increase your heart's need for blood and oxygen by raising your heart rate slowly to a predetermined level. Such a test will reveal blockage to blood flow that is only evident when the heart is stressed as it exercises. People with ischemic heart disease will often become short of breath, tired, or will have chest pain fairly quickly during a stress test. Some, however, will have no symptoms. The electrocardiogram and periodic blood pressure checks will monitor the heart's response during the stress test.

Occasionally, stress tests are performed with an injection of a radioactive dye called thallium, and an image of the heart while exercising can be seen. This is a better test for picking up coronary artery disease.

Yet another test, called an *echocardiogram,* is a painless procedure that uses ultrasound (extremely high frequency sound waves) to produce an image of the heart, and gives a clear picture of the heart's size, how it is actually functioning, and if there are any valve abnormalities or other structural changes. The test is performed by placing a transducer, a device that emits ultrasound waves, on your chest. The transducer is placed at different angles, and you are asked to change your position as well so that all parts of the heart can be seen. The image produced by the sound waves bouncing off the heart is projected onto a monitor and recorded on videotape.

Your cardiologist may recommend a *transesophageal echocardiogram,* which gives an even better, more precise image of the heart. This test is a little more involved and usually requires mild sedation. A tube with a small transducer on its tip is passed through your mouth, down your food pipe (esophagus), and into your stomach. The heart can then be viewed through the walls of the stomach.

If your doctor suspects that you have significant coronary artery disease based on the results of preliminary tests, he or she may perform *cardiac catheterization* (also called a coronary arteriogram), which determines the degree and location of the blockage. Cardiac catheterization is very common and is considered the gold standard for assessment of coronary artery disease. It generally takes about forty-five minutes to an hour and causes little discomfort.

The procedure is performed by first giving local anesthesia in the right groin region, then inserting a tube into a large artery in the groin (the femoral artery), which leads directly to the heart. A dye is injected through the tube, and an x-ray called a coronary angiogram is taken, which shows the presence or absence of coronary artery disease. Since this is an invasive test, there is a low risk (about 1 in 1,000) that it will cause serious complications, including stroke, heart attack, and death. However, overall risk varies from patient to patient and shouldn't override the potential benefits of the procedure.

Examining Your Blood

As discussed in Chapter 2, atherosclerosis is one of the leading risk factors in the development of coronary heart disease and heart attack. In order to determine your risk of atherosclerosis, your physician will probably order a blood test to measure the amount of fat circulating in your blood.

It should be noted at the start that when we talk about fat, we're usually discussing the larger category of body substances called lipids. Lipids include fats, fatty acids, sterols, and other compounds that circulate in our bloodstream and are part of our cells. Although not all lipids are fats, the two terms tend to be used interchangeably, which can be misleading. Cholesterol, for instance, is not a fat, but a fatlike lipid called a sterol.

Cholesterol is essential for a number of vital body processes, including nerve function and cell reproduction; however, there is no need for anyone to consume any cholesterol because the body manufactures all it needs. The average American, however, consumes anywhere from 600 to 1,500 milligrams of cholesterol each day, which is from two to five times the 300-milligram limit most physicians recommend.

Cholesterol travels through the bloodstream by combining with other lipids and with certain proteins; when combined these substances are called lipoproteins. It is the relationship between different kinds of lipoproteins that determines the amount of cholesterol circulating in the bloodstream.

Low-density lipoprotcins (LDL) carry about two-thirds of circulating cholesterol to the cells; this is often the "fat" we speak of when referring to the plaques that build up and cause atherosclerosis. High-density lipoproteins (HDL) carry cholesterol away from the cells to the liver, where it is eliminated from the body. We are born with about half of our cholesterol in the form of HDLs, but because the typical American diet is so high in saturated fats and cholesterol, we tend to replace HDLs with LDLs as we grow older. When you have more LDLs than HDLs, then your body is transporting more cholesterol *into* the bloodstream, which increases your risk for atherosclerosis and heart disease. If there is more LDL in your blood, you are said to have more "bad" cholesterol, since more of this fatty substance stays in the bloodstream than is eliminated. Triglycerides are another type of fat measured when testing an individual's risk for atherosclerosis.

Your doctor will discuss with you the results of your blood lipid profile. However, the National Cholesterol Education Program, sponsored by the National Institutes of Health, recommends that desirable total blood cholesterol should be below 200 mg/dl. A reading of between 200 to 239 is borderline, and any reading over 240 mg/dl is considered high. LDL cholesterol categories are as follows: less than 130 mg/dl is desirable; 130 to 159 mg/dl is borderline high; and over 160 mg/dl is high. HDL levels should range from 37 to 55. In Chapter 5, you'll learn the best ways to cut down on the amount of cholesterol you eat so that your heart and blood vessels have the best chance possible of remaining healthy and strong.

WHAT HAPPENS NEXT?

Your diagnostic workup has been completed. Your doctor has determined that you are hypertensive and/or that your heart has been affected by either hypertension or atherosclerosis. Next, together you will decide on a course of treatment that depends on several factors. Most important is the severity of the disease process. If you are moderately or severely hypertensive, your doctor may prescribe one or more antihypertensive drugs. If you have particularly high cholesterol, you may be prescribed a drug that will help lower the amount of fats circulating in your blood. If one or more of your coronary arteries shows blockage, surgery may be necessary to correct it. These drugs and surgical procedures are discussed at length in Chapter 7.

Luckily, risk factors that you can control—specifically substance abuse, diet, exercise, and stress—are the keys to cardiovascular health. But this is a lifelong proposition, one that takes dedication and awareness on your part. It also helps if you accept the help and guidance of your physician.

You and Your Doctor

Successful treatment of cardiovascular disease requires a partnership between you and your doctor, one that involves a degree of honesty and openness you may find a little uncomfortable, at least at first. Because your habits and lifestyle play such an integral role in cardiovascular health, you must feel free to tell your doctor some pretty private things about the way you lead your life.

Needless to say, then, you must trust and, to a certain extent, like your physician. This isn't to say that the two of you will become bosom buddies; your doctor must keep a certain professional distance to provide you with the best, most objective care. What it does mean, however, is that you have to feel comfortable with your doctor, and he or she with you, since the relationship between you may last for several years, perhaps for a lifetime.

If for any reason you are not happy with your current physician, you should feel free to choose another. This should not be done lightly, especially if your doctor has been caring for you and your family for a long time. On the other hand, since your medical therapy may require complex and constant adjustments, your physician should be as open to your particular needs, desires, and fears as possible. At the same time, you must be willing to accept a certain amount of responsibility for the relationship you have with your doctor. Remember, only by forming a partnership will you be able to effectively control the course of your cardiovascular health.

In order to maintain the best relationship possible with your doctor and his or her staff, the following procedures are recommended:

1. If you have high blood pressure that needs constant monitoring, ask your doctor if you can learn to take your blood pressure at home. That way, you can avoid the additional expense and time involved in an office visit. In addition, many health maintenance organizations and clinics offer blood pressure monitoring and blood testing on a walk-in basis without requiring a separate doctor's appointment.

2. One of the most common complaints among patients is the fact that they must wait extra minutes—even hours—after their scheduled appointment to see their doctor. Although such delays are often unavoidable, you may be able to cut down on your waiting time by scheduling your appointments midweek and early in the doctor's morning or afternoon schedule when he or she tends to be less

busy. Arrive on time, and remind the receptionist of your presence if you are still in the waiting room thirty minutes after your scheduled appointment.

3. Some patients feel more comfortable if they take a concerned person with them to hear the doctor's evaluation, especially if the heart or blood pressure condition is serious. Most doctors should have no objection if you decide to bring a spouse, friend, or relative with you into the office after the physical examination is complete.

4. Tell your doctor the *whole* truth; withholding facts for fear of embarrassment can easily lead to misdiagnosis or unnecessary treatment. Let your doctor know if you do not understand his or her terminology. Repeat back what your doctor says to you about diagnosis and treatment to make sure that you've understood fully what he or she has to say.

5. Cultivate a close relationship with the doctor's nurse. In most practices, the nurse is the person who will talk with you by phone in between visits.

6. If your doctor and his or her staff know you and your condition well, it may be possible for them to answer some of your questions about your medication and other health concerns over the telephone. If that is the case at your doctor's office, follow these simple rules:

- Have the phone number of your pharmacy available.
- Know the names and dosages of the drugs you take regularly.
- Protest if your call to a doctor's office is not returned in a reasonable amount of time (within a few hours or a day depending on the urgency of your concern).

That said, it really is up to you to take control of your health. If you have not yet been diagnosed with heart disease or high blood pressure, so much the better. The following chapters will help you stay healthy. If you know your cardiovascular system has been damaged, you have even more reason to follow the prescriptions set forth in Part II—even if you've been prescribed drug treatment.

IMPORTANT QUESTIONS AND ANSWERS ABOUT ESTABLISHING A MEDICAL DIAGNOSIS

Q. I sometimes get a headache and feel dizzy, especially when I'm under stress. Do these symptoms mean that my blood pressure is higher at these times than at others?

A. Not necessarily. Although headaches and dizziness are classic symptoms of hypertension, they are also symptoms of literally dozens of other conditions as well. In fact, such symptoms are experienced by far more people *without* hypertension than they are by those with high blood pressure. Moreover, having hypertension means that your blood pressure is elevated above a healthy level *most of the time,* not only when you are angry, upset, or "stressed out."

Q. My husband, a sixty-year-old smoker, had a stress test before starting an exercise program. His doctor told him he was okay. About a month later, he had a heart attack. Was the test the doctor gave him faulty?

A. Probably not. The process of atherosclerosis, which causes most heart attacks, is an uncertain one. To be large enough to measure on a stress test, an occlusion (blockage) of a heart vessel must significantly restrict the amount of oxygen the heart receives. At the time of your husband's stress test, some degree of atherosclerosis was probably present, but the vessels were clear enough to allow oxygen to feed the heart. However, during the month that followed, the artery became completely occluded, causing a heart attack.

Q. I read about a recent study that said that most angiographs are unnecessary. My doctor wants to give me one because I've been having some chest pain. Should I have one?

A. I can't answer that question without knowing your personal medical history. Research has found that more than half of all angiograms performed each year—sophisticated x-ray exams of the heart that cost a minimum of $5,000 each—are unnecessary. However, the results of this research were based on a small number of patients (about 170) and may not be applicable to the population at large. In addition, angiographs tend to be prescribed less to blacks than to whites in the first place—possibly due to racial discrimination and/or socioeconomic conditions as well as the quality of care at inner-city hospitals—so the results of this study are even more suspect for us.

It is important that you discuss your concerns with your physician and seek a second opinion if you continue to have any doubts. If you decide to obtain a second opinion, it is important that you do so quickly; often, the need for an angiogram is immediate and to delay the test may put you at increased risk for a heart attack or other serious conditions.

Part II

Preventing Cardiovascular Disease

CHAPTER 4

Coming to Terms with Substance Abuse

Walk through almost any African-American neighborhood and you'll probably see more ads for cigarettes and liquor than for any other products. Beautiful models with cigarettes in their hands smile and tell us that smoking is sophisticated and glamorous—a habit of the beautiful and healthy. Malt liquor is equated with the power of tigers, beer with the purity of mountain springs, and brandy with smooth seduction. Although no ads proclaim the virtue of cocaine, the drug remains stubbornly alluring to many young black Americans, especially those who consider themselves without hope in a country that has for so long ignored them.

It isn't difficult to be drawn into substance abuse, and many of us are. Smoking, drinking, and drug abuse remain epidemic throughout the United States, in small towns as well as large cities. It appears, however, that these habits are more firmly entrenched and affect more people in the poorer black communities of the inner cities than anywhere else.

There are many reasons why substance abuse affects proportionately more black than white Americans. At least part of the responsibility lies with the above-described advertising strategies used by the cigarette and liquor companies to market their products specifically to blacks. Altogether, the tobacco industry spends more than $2 billion a year promoting cigarettes and a higher and higher percentage of that money is being spent in African-American neighborhoods every year.

Even more important is the fact that more blacks than whites live under conditions bound to induce stress— high-crime neighborhoods, periods of prolonged unemployment, reduced expectations and opportunities— which they hope to relieve with a cigarette, a drink, or a hit of cocaine. Unfortunately, the psychological and physical effects of substance abuse result in anything *but* relaxation.

Cigarettes, alcohol, and illicit drugs may be addictive, which means that many people develop both a psychological and a physical craving for them—even when they no longer derive any pleasure from the habit. The nicotine in tobacco, for instance, is an addictive drug: smokers feel that they can relieve their addiction only by smoking another cigarette. Many smokers crave cigarettes during times of special stress—how many of you reach for a cigarette when you're nervous or angry?— which tells us that smokers have psychological as well as physical needs they expect cigarettes to meet. Over time, the need for cigarettes, alcohol, and/or drugs may completely overwhelm the addict so that nothing—including solid medical evidence that the habit is likely to cause serious disease and/or death—is more important than relieving that need.

It must be recognized here that not everyone who partakes of cigarettes, alcohol, or illicit drugs automatically becomes addicted. An individual's susceptibility to a particular substance depends on a variety of factors, including heredity, physiology, and psychological makeup. However, it also must be stressed that those who abuse certain substances put themselves at serious risk for several life-threatening diseases as long as they involve themselves in these bad habits.

In addition to being a major risk factor for the development of heart disease, for instance, smoking also leads to emphysema, lung cancer, throat and mouth cancer, and a host of gastrointestinal and central nervous system disorders as well. Alcohol abuse, also a major risk factor for cardiovascular disease, can eventually lead to cirrhosis of the liver, pancreatic disease, severe gastritis, and a host of neurological disorders. Illicit drugs, especially cocaine, can result in devastating psychological and physical addiction, sudden death from cardiac complications, and, if injected carelessly, the spread of AIDS (acquired immune deficiency syndrome) and other infectious diseases.

In this chapter, we'll discuss the three types of addictive substances commonly abused by black (as well as white) Americans—cigarettes, alcohol, and illicit drugs, specifically cocaine—how they affect the human body, specifically the cardiovascular system, and the best ways to rid yourself of the habit.

SMOKING AND YOUR CARDIOVASCULAR SYSTEM

According to the United States Surgeon General, cigarette smoking is the single most preventable cause of heart disease and is responsible for nearly 20 percent of all heart-disease related deaths annually. Each year nearly half a million American smokers die prematurely of a smoking-related disease. Smokers are three times more likely to die of cancer than nonsmokers. The Framingham Heart Study found that men who smoke have a tenfold increased risk of death from cardiac arrest over those men who do not smoke. Among women smokers, the mortality rate is fivefold over women nonsmokers.

Although some statistics show that black smokers tend to smoke fewer cigarettes per day than white smokers (ten to twenty cigarettes per day among blacks compared with twenty to thirty per day among whites), overall smoking prevalence is much higher among blacks than whites, especially among black males. As of 1994, 34 percent of black men and 22 percent of black women smoke, compared to 29 percent of white men and 25 percent of white women.

For both blacks and whites, the dangers from cigarette smoke start with just one cigarette a day and increase with every cigarette smoked: smoking one to ten cigarettes per day doubles the mortality rate from heart disease, smoking ten to twenty cigarettes per day increases the mortality *another* 25 percent, and smoking more than two packs a day triples the death rate. Smokers have a stunning 70 percent higher rate of death from heart disease than nonsmokers. Women who smoke seem to be even more at risk of dying from heart disease. Smoking appears to lower the normal level of the female hormone estrogen, a substance believed to help prevent heart disease.

Among both males and females, the combination of cigarette smoking and hypertension—an all-too-common combination among African-Americans—is especially lethal. Black or white, male or female, if you know you have a predisposition to hypertension and you smoke cigarettes, you've increased your risk for having a fatal heart attack by many times.

Not only does smoking directly affect the cardiovascular system, but most people who smoke also tend to have a number of other bad habits that can increase their risks for developing atherosclerosis, hypertension, and coronary heart disease. As you've probably noticed among your friends and family, those who smoke are also more likely to eat poorly and drink heavily, and less likely to exercise regularly than those who don't smoke. As a rule, then, smokers tend to take more risks with their cardiovascular system than nonsmokers.

How Smoking Affects Your Cardiovascular System

There are some four thousand substances identified in cigarette smoke—some highly toxic and carcinogenic (cancer-causing). Nicotine is cigarette smoke's main ingredient. When you inhale a cigarette, nicotine immediately enters the bloodstream and reaches the brain within six seconds, where more than 15 percent of it is absorbed. Nicotine is a stimulant; when it reaches the brain, it signals the adrenal glands to release norepinephrine and epinephrine (adrenaline), which increases both the systolic and diastolic pressure. Your heart beats faster, it pumps more blood, and your arteries work harder to push the blood through your body.

In addition to directly causing an increase in heart and vessel activity, cigarette smoking also contributes to the acceleration of atherosclerosis. Nicotine, as well as other products of cigarette smoke, raises the amount of fats and cholesterol circulating in the bloodstream, which form plaque on artery walls. In fact, cigarette smoking has been shown to raise the level of low-density lipoproteins or LDLs (the "bad" cholesterol) by as much as 10 percent. Atherosclerosis is accelerated by another ingredient of cigarette smoke, carbon monoxide, as well. Carbon monoxide damages the cells that form the inner linings of arterial walls, making them more susceptible to plaque buildup.

To make matters worse, carbon monoxide is carried through the bloodstream by the same blood component, hemoglobin, that transports oxygen. The more carbon monoxide in the bloodstream, therefore, the less oxygen is being carried to the vital organs, including the heart. Therefore, at the same time that nicotine is stimulating heart and vessel activity, carbon monoxide prevents oxygen from helping the body do this extra work. Over time, this extra stress weakens both heart and vessel walls and further paves the way for atherosclerosis and hemorrhage.

Cigarette smoking also causes chemical changes in the blood itself, causing it to become more viscous, or sticky, which results in the formation of large blood clots, a process called thrombosis. As you'll see more clearly after reading Chapter 9, these clots can cause both strokes and heart attacks.

Take the Good News to Heart

Since the dangers of smoking were made public by the Surgeon General in 1964, almost 50 million people have stopped smoking for good. The fact that so many people no longer smoke accounts for at least part of the remarkable decrease in the number of cardiovascular deaths in the last two decades. Unfortunately, a smaller proportion of blacks than whites have chosen to stop smoking during this same period and a larger proportion of young blacks, especially young black women, have chosen to start.

The good news is that smokers of any race who quit will reduce their risks of having a heart attack to the same level as those people who have never smoked at all. Indeed, there is ample evidence that within just two years after quitting, ex-smokers will have cut their risks of having fatal heart attacks in half, and after ten years, their risk will be no higher than that of nonsmokers.

Though it takes a long time for such benefits of quitting to be realized, other improvements are experienced almost immediately. Althea W., a smoker who quit the habit after smoking for more than thirty years, reported to me that she felt she was able to taste food in a whole new way. Other patients report having more energy, fresher breath, whiter teeth, and a sense of clear-headedness that they hadn't experienced since they began smoking.

In my experience, savoring these changes, even if they may seem unimportant or cosmetic, will go a long way to help bolster a patient's commitment to quit the habit. And the longer someone goes without smoking, the less likely it will be that he or she will start again.

Ways to Stop Smoking

We smoke for many reasons—some people say smoking calms them down, some say it picks them up. Some like the way smoking makes them look, thinking it gives them a sophisticated, powerful image. Some people smoke when they're anxious, some when alone, some only at parties. But all smokers have one thing in common: All of them are contributing to the likelihood that they will develop heart disease—especially if they also have hypertension.

In some ways, it has never been easier to quit smoking than it is today, mainly because the nature of addiction is better understood than ever before. Today, however, there are a number of effective means of quitting and most of them have few, if any side effects.

Cold Turkey There are those who like or need to feel in control of their lives, and smoking, with its cravings and almost slavish obsession with finding and smoking a cigarette, undermines that sense of control. In fact, some smokers choose to quit in large part so that they can reestablish their sense of self-control. These people are often the ones who can quit without first gaining medical help or emotional support for their decision; they simply don't pick up or light another cigarette, a method of quitting known as "cold turkey."

They may do so after having a scare, such as experiencing shortness of breath while walking up the stairs, developing chest pains after exertion, or even having a heart attack. Or they may simply wake up one morning and decide that they may no longer want to smoke. A friend of mine once told me that he caught a glimpse of himself smoking while walking past a window one day, and decided that he simply didn't see himself as a smoker. It was almost as if he didn't recognize the smoker he saw in the reflection. So he quit on the spot.

There are people who have the inner resources to do this, but most of us don't. If you decide to try to quit this way, you may find some support by calling your local American Lung Association and/or American Heart Association and asking for one of the many publications (see Resources for more information). Quitting cold turkey is extremely difficult, mainly because the physical effects of withdrawing from nicotine—irritability, insomnia, loss of appetite, headaches, coughing, and mood swings—are often quite disturbing. If you can do it, quitting this way can give you a profound sense of accomplishment. On the other hand, however, failing may leave you feeling extremely discouraged. For this reason, quitting cold turkey is probably not the best way to stop smoking. Instead, choose a method that offers you some medical and/or social support.

Hypnosis and Behavior Modification   Among the popular alternatives for smoking cessation are hypnosis and behavior modification. In successful hypnosis, a sleeplike state is induced by a trained professional who then makes a hypnotic suggestion that you will no longer want to smoke. When you are again fully awake, you most likely will not want to smoke—at least for a time. Often, however, the effects of hypnosis last only a few hours or days, not the weeks it may take an individual to withdraw from nicotine and the other aspects of cigarette addiction.

Behavior modification, on the other hand, seeks to change one's behavior over the long term. There are several types of behavior modification, including aversive counter-conditioning. This relatively effective technique aims to get the smoker to equate smoking with a negative response. This is achieved by pairing smoking with a negative stimulus, like a mild electric shock or a drug that produces nausea. In the first instance, a mild electric shock would be administered each time you inhaled a cigarette. Eventually, smoking becomes a negative event for you, and you will want to quit.

If this approach seems rather drastic, it is. There are other, less overwhelming forms of behavior modification. One such method involves keeping a log of when you smoke in order to find out why you smoke when you do. Once you know why you smoke, you can begin to change those things that make you want a cigarette. For instance, you may find that you always reach for a cigarette after meeting with your boss; after you quit, you'll want to replace smoking with another stress-relieving action, such as taking a short walk or drinking a cup of tea.

If you are interested in hypnosis and/or behavior modification methods for stopping smoking, ask your physician to recommend a reputable hypnotist or therapist.

Stop-Smoking Clinics There are a number of stop-smoking clinics and they vary in their approach to getting people to quit. Most use some combination of behavior modification, relaxation, and self-awareness exercises and all stress the importance of group support: the "we're all in this together" feeling seems to help many people kick the habit. Your local American Heart Association will be able to direct you to the clinic nearest you.

Nicotine Gum and Nicotine Patches Nicotine gum and nicotine patches, which are now available over-the-counter at drugstores, work by releasing nicotine, the addictive substance in cigarette smoke, into the bloodstream in an effort to help smokers break the habit of smoking without experiencing extreme withdrawal symptoms. Using these methods, smokers gradually reduce the amount of their nicotine intake until they are weaned from it completely.

The nicotine patch, is applied to the upper arm with a self-sticking adhesive. The patch releases a steady amount of nicotine into the bloodstream continuously. They come in two or three dosages of nicotine, and heavy smokers are usually started on the highest dosage. The dosage is then reduced every few weeks until the patient can be weaned off nicotine completely.

The patch seems to be preferable to gum for several reasons. Many potential ex-smokers report that nicotine gum causes irritation of the mouth and throat, bad breath, and stained teeth. These factors reduce patient compliance with the gum regimen. Also, the amount of nicotine release varies with the number of sticks of gum chewed and the length of time they are chewed. If the level of nicotine in the bloodstream isn't high enough, the craving for a cigarette may return.

The main adverse effect of the nicotine patch is skin irritation under and around the area where the patch is applied. Patients are also warned not to smoke at all while on the patch, as the level of nicotine in your blood would be extremely high and could cause coronary artery spasms and increase the risk of heart attacks.

The use of nicotine substitutes is most successful when accompanied by a behavior modification program of some kind to help smokers overcome their psychological as well as physical addiction to smoking.

Sticking to It

Despite the advances made in recent years, the strongest determinant of your success in quitting smoking will be your personality type and the strength of your desire to quit. Like exercise or dieting, becoming a nonsmoker takes time and energy. The first three months—before not smoking becomes as much a part of your life as smoking had been—are often the toughest. It is during this time that most ex-smokers start smoking again, especially if other stresses in life, like a divorce or difficulties at work, intrude.

There's no way around the bad news: Recidivism rates among smokers are quite high indeed. If you're a smoker, you may have already tried to quit many times before. To help you stick to your resolve to quit for good this time, I offer you these hints to make your struggle to stop smoking a little easier to bear.

List Your Reasons for Quitting Write down why you want to stop smoking and keep the list available so that you can refer to it when your commitment wanes. Be as specific as possible: "I don't want my kids to see me and think it's all right for them to start;" "I'm sick of not really tasting my grandmother's good cooking;" "My husband thinks my breath smells bad;" "My doctor says my heart is getting weaker every day."

Get Your Friends and Family to Help You Social support is extremely important to anyone trying to break a bad habit. Don't be afraid to ask your friends and family not to smoke in front of you, or to keep you busy so you don't want to smoke. You might be surprised at how many find the courage to stop themselves just by watching you.

Keep Low-Calorie Snack Foods Handy Simply having something in your mouth—other than a cigarette!—may help you break the habit. Unsalted, unbuttered popcorn, sugarless candy and gum, fresh vegetables and fruit are all healthy alternatives.

Change Your Routine Many people smoke after every meal or when the telephone rings or whenever they have an alcoholic beverage, and it is at those times when quitting seems most difficult. In those cases, it is important to replace one habit—lighting up—with another. Instead of smoking after meals, for instance, get up from the table, brush your teeth, then go for a walk. Just getting up from the table will help; if you brush your teeth, you'll be less likely to "dirty" them again with cigarette smoke; walking will take your mind off your craving for nicotine.

Go Where It Is Impossible to Smoke These days it's getting easier and easier to find public places where smoking simply isn't allowed. Museums, department stores, concert halls, and movie theaters are just a few of the pleasant places you can spend time where you won't be tempted to light up. Catch a movie, volunteer at a church supper, window-shop in a smoke-free mall—go anyplace where you can't smoke but where you'll still enjoy yourself. Today, almost all restaurants have nonsmoking sections; treat yourself to a special lunch or dinner—just make sure you sit where smoking a cigarette is impossible.

Whenever Possible, Take Public Transportation For many people, smoking while driving is an ingrained habit. If that's true for you, take public transportation as often as possible. Luckily, many African-Americans live in urban areas, where buses and subways are common. Not only is most public transportation off limits to smoking, but you'll be freeing yourself from another situation—driving—in which you might be tempted to smoke.

Create a "Smoke-Free" Environment Ever smell your clothes after you've worn them all day while you were smoking? Does your furniture have a stale odor to it? Once you've decided to stop smoking, wash and press your entire wardrobe, throw out every ashtray, and if possible, have your carpet and upholstery cleaned. You'll notice immediately how fresh your clothes and furniture smell and how much more beautiful a house without ashes and ashtrays can be.

Increase Your Exercise Not only will exercise help you minimize any potential weight gain, but you'll feel better almost immediately from the effects of exercise on your entire body. Many people find that exercise relieves stress—one of the main reasons they started to smoke in the first place.

Does Quitting Smoking Mean Gaining Weight?

One of the most common questions about quitting smoking involves how it will affect one's weight. Since many African-Americans, especially black women, are already large—and obesity is itself an important risk factor for cardiovascular disease—the question is a good one to ask.

Unfortunately, it is true that many people turn to food

as a substitute for cigarettes and gain a few pounds. The oral gratification aspect of smoking—simply enjoying having something in your mouth—may cause you to turn to food when you no longer can reach for a cigarette. In addition, your metabolism—the rate at which you use energy—may slow down a bit when you quit smoking; you may find yourself not able to eat quite as much as you could while smoking without gaining some weight.

Does all this mean you shouldn't stop smoking? Not at all. First of all, studies have shown that the average weight gain in an ex-smoker is only 5 to 10 pounds, and some of this weight gain may be caused by increased fluid retention during the withdrawal period and hence is only temporary. Second, giving up cigarettes is far healthier for you than adding a few extra pounds. In fact, according to the American Heart Association, it would take the addition of about 75 to 100 pounds to negate the health benefits that a normal smoker gains by quitting.

A more positive factor in an ex-smoker's potential weight gain is the brand new sense of taste that goes along with quitting smoking. Ex-smokers often remark on how good food tastes when the nicotine and other chemicals no longer dull the taste buds. This can work to your advantage, however, when you rediscover how delicious fresh (and low-calorie/low-fat) fruits and vegetables really taste. (Read more about a healthy diet in Chapter 6.)

Although quitting smoking will not be easy for you, it is the single most positive step you can take to improve the health and strength of your cardiovascular system.

ALCOHOL AND YOUR CARDIOVASCULAR SYSTEM

To help cope with the incredible social and financial stresses faced by most black Americans, an alarming number of us turn to alcohol. Alcohol is actually a drug, the most common and pervasive in the world. It is a sedative designed to relax the central nervous system. Taken occasionally and in moderate quantities, alcohol can indeed provide pleasure and relaxation. However, among both black and white Americans, alcohol can also be an addictive, life-threatening substance.

After tobacco, alcohol abuse is the leading cause of premature death in America and is associated with the loss of more than 100,000 lives annually, many of them on the nation's highways.

Studies have shown that even moderate drinkers run an increased risk of breast cancer and heavy drinkers have high rates of liver disease; in fact, alcoholics who continue to drink decrease their life expectancy by ten to fifteen years. Lost employment and productivity due to drinking costs approximately $70 billion annually and this lost revenue especially affects the already disadvantaged black communities.

As anyone who has experienced a hangover can tell you, alcohol taken in large doses is toxic to the human body. Although the headache, nausea, and dizziness related to a hangover is short-lived, over the long term, alcohol abuse may cause cirrhosis of the liver, gastrointestinal conditions, and neurological disorders, as well as cardiac problems.

When alcohol enters the body, it is absorbed directly through the stomach and small intestine into the bloodstream and then into every part of the body that contains water, including major organs like the brain, lungs, kidneys, and heart, and distributes itself equally both inside and outside of cells. Only about 5 percent of the alcohol is eliminated from the body through breath, urine, or sweat; the rest is broken down by the liver. It takes the liver about three hours to break down the alcohol consumed in less than one ounce of whiskey.

Within a few minutes of ingestion, alcohol reaches the brain. Its initial effect on brain cells is stimulation, which accounts for the "buzz" many people feel after a drink or two. Alcohol also acts to depress those brain functions related to inhibition and judgment, which causes most drinkers to feel friendlier and more gregarious, at least for a time. The flip side of this release from natural personality constraints are the mood swings and crying jags experienced by many drinkers. Judgment, memory, and sensory perception are all progressively impaired as the level of alcohol in the bloodstream rises.

As well as affecting mood, alcohol decreases motor ability, muscle function, and eyesight coordination. Respiratory function, heart rate, and circulation also slow down. Severe alcohol poisoning results in death when so much alcohol is consumed that the central nervous system shuts down, causing the lungs and heart to stop functioning.

Most people, however, experience only mild and temporary ill effects from alcohol. The major health problems associated with alcohol—apart from those caused by drunk driving—occur in individuals who drink heavily on a regular basis over an extended period of time or those who indulge in binge drinking. People who drink alcohol in these ways are almost always addicted to the substance, a condition known as alcoholism. Later in this chapter, you'll learn how to recognize some of the signs of alcoholism and where you can turn for help if you or someone you love has a drinking problem. In the meantime, let's look at the effects alcohol has on your cardiovascular system.

The French Paradox

Amid all the gloom and doom about the dangers of alcohol, there is a bit of good news for moderate, occasional drinkers—and there are millions of us. Indeed, moderate drinking—defined as two ounces of one hundred proof alcohol a day, the equivalent of about two beers or one four-ounce glass of wine—may actually have *beneficial* effects on the cardiovascular system. This phenomenon has been nicknamed the "French paradox" because the health benefits of alcohol consumption are especially evident among the French, who have far lower mortality rates due to heart disease than Americans—despite the fact that they eat a diet equal or higher in fat levels.

The difference between the American and French diets appears to be in the amount of alcohol—specifically red wine—the two cultures imbibe. Red wine apparently affects the cardiovascular system by working to increase the levels of HDL, the "good" cholesterol. By what mechanism this occurs is still not completely understood, but scientists believe that the phenols that are present in some alcoholic beverages, work as antioxidants to help metabolize lipids and more quickly remove them from the bloodstream.

Studies show that the benefits to the cardiovascular system derived from moderate alcohol consumption affects black Americans in the same way. Therefore, if you enjoy a cocktail before dinner or a glass of wine with your meal, feel free to continue this pleasurable and apparently harmless habit. However, if you are unable to handle alcohol physically or emotionally, if you have a family history of alcoholism, or if you simply don't like to drink, the risks of alcoholism far outweigh the benefits and you should not feel pressured to partake.

As consumption of alcohol progresses beyond two drinks a day, so do the risks to health. As already stated, heavy drinking damages almost every part of the body, including your heart and blood vessels.

Alcohol and Hypertension

The relationship between heavy drinking—again, more than two or three drinks a day—and hypertension has been well documented. Several studies, including the Framingham Heart Study, the Los Angeles Heart Study, and the Chicago Western Electric Study, showed that patients who have histories of long-term, heavy drinking had significantly higher blood pressures than those patients who were light drinkers or abstainers. Although these studies focused on mostly white patients, a 1968 report that used about 12,730 black subjects confirmed the link. In this report, called the Kaiser-Permanente Multiphasic Health Examination Study, researchers found that the higher a person's daily alcohol intake, the higher their blood pressure. They also noted that among white men and women, blood pressure was consistently higher after three drinks per day.

In this study, the relationship between alcohol intake and hypertension was not as strong in blacks as it was in whites, though blood pressure was still significantly higher after three drinks a day.

This study also showed that patients who consumed one to two drinks per day had slightly lower blood pressures than those patients who abstained from drinking at all, which suggests that moderate alcohol intake may have a favorable effect on blood pressure. The more alcohol a patient consumes after the first or second drink, however, the more he or she risks damaging his cardiovascular system.

One of my patients, a sixty-year-old African-American man whom I treated for high blood pressure at a Veterans Administration hospital, had been drinking a quart of whiskey a day and saw no reason to quit. As Hank J. saw it, he had no major health problems. He didn't have cirrhosis of the liver, and he didn't understand that his heavy drinking and his hypertension were linked. Before he stopped drinking, his high blood pressure was quite difficult to control and required high dosages of antihypertension medication. Once I got him to see this connection and understand the dangers of high blood pressure, Hank decided to quit. After three months of not drinking, he was able to significantly lower the amount of medication he takes on a daily basis.

If you have high blood pressure, it is best that you keep your drinking to a minimum. In addition to its direct effects on the blood pressure system, alcohol interacts poorly with many antihypertensive medications. If you are taking medication, make sure you discuss drinking alcohol with your doctor.

Alcohol and Stroke

The exact relationship between drinking and stroke is unknown, though it is thought that increased blood pressure due to heavy drinking contributes to the risk of a particularly devastating type of stroke, called hemorrhagic stroke. In a hemorrhagic stroke, blood vessels in the brain weakened by years of hypertension suddenly burst, flooding the brain with blood and destroying brain tissue. One particularly tragic story of a stroke associated with drinking was that of a thirty-six-year-old African-American mother of three, who was suffering from alcoholism and hypertension. She had originally been referred to me because of her poorly controlled hypertension. On one particular visit, I tried to get her to consider a rehabilitation program, but she refused. About two months later, she had a massive hemorrhagic stroke, presumably caused by her uncontrolled hypertension complicated by alcoholism.

Alcohol and Dilated Cardiomyopathy

In a small number of cases, heavy drinking over a long period of time may directly damage the heart, causing a condition known as cardiomyopathy. Heart muscle cells are destroyed both by alcohol itself and by the nutritional deficiencies that often occur when alcohol is the drinker's main source of caloric intake. With heart muscle destruction, the heart becomes so baggy and inelastic that it can no longer pump enough blood to the rest of the body.

Alcohol and Cardiac Arrhythmias

Another possible effect of heavy drinking is cardiac arrhythmias, or irregular heartbeats. Alcohol is thought to provoke arrhythmias by stimulating the sympathetic nervous system; in fact, alcoholics tend to have higher blood levels of the "fight-or-flight" hormones, epinephrine and norepinephrine. Acute arrythmia is especially common among binge drinkers—those with a history of heavy but sporadic drinking. It is also called "holiday heart syndrome" because it frequently occurs during holidays when you drink much more than usual in a relatively short period of time. Arrhythmias can be easily controlled or eliminated by cutting down on alcohol, and they are an acute rather than a long-term effect of heavy drinking.

How Much Is Too Much?

Although alcohol is a drug, its use is legally and socially sanctioned and therefore a strict definition of alcoholism is difficult to come by. According to the National Institute on Alcohol Abuse and Alcoholism, a person who averages more than two drinks a day can be considered a heavy drinker; someone who craves alcohol even when the substance interferes with day-to-day living and poses severe health risks may be considered an alcoholic.

Alcohol problems occur at all educational and social levels, in every age group, among both men and women, and in both the African-American and white populations. Unfortunately, it isn't always easy to tell when someone—even when that someone is you—has crossed the line between moderate drinking and alcoholism. Many people drink secretly and are able to hold down a job, attend church, even keep up appearances in front of neighbors and friends. Nevertheless, once you feel that you've lost control over alcohol, it is likely that it has harmed both your personal emotional life and your health.

If you think you have a problem with alcohol, ask yourself the following questions. If the answer to any of them is yes, you may want to consider getting some help.

- Do you drink—or crave a drink—when you feel under pressure at work or at home?

- Do you argue with friends or family over your drinking habits?
- Have you ever injured yourself or another person while drinking?
- Do you find yourself forcing yourself to go "on the wagon" often?
- Has alcohol ever caused you to miss work?
- Have you ever "blacked out" or been unable to remember what happened while you were drinking?

As in most things, then, the lesson about alcohol is "everything in moderation." Will one or two drinks now and then hurt you? Probably not, and in fact, moderate drinking may even do you some good. Remember, however, the more you drink, the more you put your life on the line.

COCAINE AND YOUR CARDIOVASCULAR SYSTEM

- Acute myocardial infarction (heart attack)
- Myocardial ischemia (lack of blood flow to heart tissue)
- Cardiac arrhythmias (irregular heartbeats)
- Pulmonary edema (fluid in lungs usually caused by heart failure)
- Stroke

This abbreviated list of the life-threatening medical emergencies related to the use of cocaine should be enough to make anyone think twice about using this illegal and highly dangerous drug. Unfortunately, we know from our local newspapers, and perhaps from painful personal experience, that drugs—particularly cocaine and its derivatives—are a scourge in far too many African-American communities. Indeed, our young people, especially our young men, are dying in record numbers because of cocaine's grip on our neighborhoods. If not shot to death by increasingly ruthless drug dealers, black youth are brought to hospital emergency rooms or city morgues after being felled by heart attacks or strokes.

Cocaine is derived from the leaves of the coca bush, which grows primarily in the Andes of South America, and has been used for centuries for medicinal, religious, and other purposes. In recent years, there has been a dramatic increase in the "recreational" use of the drug, which can be snorted into the nose, injected intravenously, or smoked. No matter how it is ingested, cocaine produces an intense, but short-lived, feeling of euphoria and energy that lasts about twenty to thirty minutes. When the drug wears off, however, these temporary pleasurable sensations are replaced by two things: a low feeling of depression and a craving for more of the drug.

In any form, cocaine raises the breathing rate, heart rate, blood pressure, and body temperature. By causing the coronary arteries to constrict, blood pressure rises and the blood supply to the heart is diminished, which can result in heart attacks or convulsions. It may also make blood cells called platelets more likely to clump together and form blood clots that cause heart attacks. In addition, cocaine's effects on the nervous system disrupt the normal rhythm of the heart, causing arrhythmias, or abnormal heartbeats.

Crack cocaine, which was first introduced to the United States in the mid-1980s, is perhaps the most dangerous form of cocaine. Smoking cocaine allows more of the harmful substance to reach the brain in larger and more concentrated doses than when the drug is either injected or snorted. Therefore, crack is even more likely than other forms of cocaine to cause coma, convulsions, and death. Crack is also extremely addictive, one of the most addictive substances known to man.

Because of the unique way that cocaine works on the heart and nervous system, drug users need not be addicts to be at risk. In fact, even in the absence of any underlying illness or heart disease, a single use of only a small amount of the drug has been known to be fatal. Unlike the advice given in this text and elsewhere about the feasibility of moderate alcohol use, cocaine in all its forms should be avoided at all costs by everyone, regardless of race, sex, or age.

The lack of federally funded treatment centers and prevention programs has only exacerbated the problems faced by poor black addicts and their families. Successful treatment of cocaine addiction consists of first detoxifying the body of the drug, which can be quite painful, then intense psychotherapy and group support. The best venue for such treatment is in a private clinic specializing in addiction therapy; unfortunately, spaces in these clinics are both limited and often prohibitively expensive. Currently, there are only a few free self-help programs, such as Cocaine Anonymous, and low-cost clinics available to help addicts and their families break free from the stranglehold of cocaine addiction.

As stated at the beginning of this chapter, a larger proportion of black than white Americans smoke cigarettes, drink alcohol, and use cocaine. A variety of factors are responsible for this fact, one of the most important being that more blacks than whites live under stressful conditions—high-crime neighborhoods, lack of economic opportunity—complicated by the enduring scourge of racism. In the next chapter, you'll learn how stress itself affects the cardiovascular system and find out how to alleviate at least some of the tension you may be feeling on a day-to-day basis.

IMPORTANT QUESTIONS AND ANSWERS ABOUT COMING TO TERMS WITH SUBSTANCE ABUSE

Q. I'm a fifty-two-year-old woman who was a two-pack a day smoker until about three years ago when I quit cold turkey. Today, I smoke about three or four cigarettes a

day, usually one after every meal when I still get a craving for a smoke. Even though I still smoke a little, haven't I done something to help improve my health?

A. Absolutely. The health hazards from cigarettes stem from the amount of tar, nicotine, and other deadly chemicals you inhale—that's why filters that reduce the amount of tar inhaled are *slightly* better for you than unfiltered cigarettes. Therefore, the less you smoke, the better. However, if you are really able to smoke just three cigarettes a day, you are one of the extremely rare individuals who can control this insidious habit. I would suggest that you attempt to quit altogether so that you don't find that three cigarettes a day creeping up to four, then five, then a full-blown two-pack a day habit.

Q. My father was an alcoholic and now my older brother is in a recovery program to help him stop drinking. Is alcoholism inherited? I'm only eighteen, but should I be worried that I might become an alcoholic, too?

A. It appears that at least a *tendency* toward alcoholism may be genetically determined. Studies show that children of alcoholics are three to four times more likely to become alcoholics than children of nonalcoholic parents. Moreover, studies among twins show that identical twins (who inherit the exact same genes) of an alcoholic parent are twice as likely to become alcoholics as nonidentical twins. However, alcoholism, like hypertension and heart disease, is a *multifactorial* disease: it involves both genetic and environmental factors. The child of an alcoholic parent is no more *doomed* to have a drinking problem than the child of a heart patient is *doomed* to suffer a heart attack. The fact that such a problem exists in a family, however, should not be ignored. If you are worried about the way drinking might affect you, you should seriously consider choosing not to drink at all.

Q. My twenty-one-year-old son was a big fan of Len Bias, the basketball star who died suddenly of a cocaine-

related heart attack. My son insists that Mr. Bias must have been an addict and that occasional use of cocaine isn't that harmful. Is that true?

A. Unfortunately—and most emphatically—your son is under a terribly misguided though popular misconception. Len Bias was not a cocaine addict; in fact, there is evidence that this incident was the first time he had used cocaine. Cocaine reacts very unpredictably in the brain and on the heart, and although cases of sudden death are relatively rare, they do occur. The amount of cocaine one individual can tolerate at a particular time is highly variable and completely unpredictable. In addition, cocaine—especially crack cocaine—is highly addictive. Anecdotal evidence indicates that crack smokers can become psychologically and physically addicted after just one experience with the drug. Cocaine is very risky business indeed.

CHAPTER 5

Coping with Stress

Thomas K., a forty-year-old patient of mine, has worked as a paralegal in a downtown corporate law firm for more than eight years. His job is a demanding one: he works on strict deadlines for high-powered attorneys and frequently must put in overtime on evenings and weekends. He hasn't had a vacation in about two years.

Although Thomas has performed his job well and received favorable evaluations, he has been promoted just once. He claims that his white colleagues, on the other hand, receive more rotations to higher-profile, higher-paying positions even though they do equal or even slightly less excellent work than does he. Thomas admits that his superiors have always been cordial to him and that no overt displays of racism have occurred. Because the signs of discrimination are so subtle, Thomas feels unable to express the anger and hostility he feels toward both his co-workers and his bosses, partly because they may be misplaced (perhaps his work *isn't* as good as he thinks) and partly because he is afraid he'll lose his job if he speaks up.

I first met Thomas last year, after he had suffered a mild heart attack probably related to his hypertension (his reading upon my first exam was 165/100). As discussed in Chapter 2, it is impossible in most cases to assign a specific cause to the development of hypertension;

there are several things related to diet, exercise, and family history that have an impact on blood pressure. Indeed, Thomas himself had a few risk factors for hypertension, including the fact that he was about 10 pounds overweight and did not exercise very often. However, I believe that at least part of the reason Thomas has high blood pressure today is the amount of stress he experiences on the job every day.

There is no doubt that stress causes physical reactions: just think of how your heart races and pounds and how the hairs on the back of your neck stand up when you are truly frightened, or how your stomach drops and your mouth goes dry when you see the person you love. The problem in making a direct link between stress and health, however, is problematic. First, except for extreme situations, such as the death of a spouse, a clear definition of stress does not exist. In addition, we tend to forget that stress can be physical as well as emotional—your body experiences stress every time you mow the lawn or carry a sack of groceries up a flight of stairs. And stress is positive as well as negative. The emotions attached to the birth of a child may create as much stress as the death of someone close to you.

Second, not everyone responds to stress in the same way; some people yell and scream at the drop of a hat, while others never blink an eye even when disaster occurs. But it could be that the outwardly calm person is seething inside, driving blood pressure to even higher levels than the person who openly expresses anger, frustration, and/or panic. Indeed, as we'll discuss later in this chapter, *how* you cope with stress matters as much as how *much* stress exists in your life.

THE PHYSIOLOGY OF STRESS

A brief description of the nervous system might be helpful in understanding the effect of stress on the body, and thus on hypertension and heart disease. The nervous system is divided into two major components: the central and the peripheral nervous systems. The brain and the spinal cord comprise the central nervous system, while the peripheral nervous system consists of bundles of nerves radiating from the spinal cord to all other parts of the body. The peripheral nervous system is further divided into the somatic nervous system, which controls voluntary muscles like your biceps or hamstrings; and the autonomic nervous system, which governs the glands and the involuntary muscles of the internal organs, like the heart.

There is one more level of division within the nervous system: the autonomic nervous system is split into the parasympathetic division, which maintains the routine bodily functions like digestion and breathing; and the sympathetic division, which functions as the arousal center during emergencies or stressful situations.

It is the sympathetic division of your autonomic nervous system that affects your cardiovascular system. It triggers such bodily reactions as increased heart rate, sweating, faster and shallower breathing, and increased blood pressure. These reactions, as we discussed in Chapter 2, are triggered by hormones (epinephrine and norepinephrine) released when danger or stress is sensed by the brain. The job of these hormones is to stimulate heart and blood vessel action, in effect preparing the body for a physical fight against the perceived stress. If your sympathetic nervous system is stimulated to prompt these reactions steadily over a long time, your blood pressure may become elevated on a permanent basis, a condition we know of as hypertension.

Stress Among African-Americans

All human beings, regardless of their race or socioeconomic status, face stress in one form or another. Even those people who appear to have everything they need to enjoy a calm and easy life, such as money, a good education, and a loving family, may develop stress-related illnesses, including stomach ulcers, headaches, and hypertension.

Nevertheless, there is no doubt that conditions in low-income, inner-city neighborhoods are especially likely to induce long-term anxiety among their inhabitants, a disproportionate number of whom are African-Americans. Unemployment, exposure to gang warfare and other violent crime, constant financial worries, and overcrowded or substandard housing are all problems that affect far too many African-Americans. Given these factors, more cases of hypertension caused or exacerbated by chronic stress are likely to occur among the black population, helping to explain at least some of the disparity between the rates of hypertension in the black and white communities.

Another important factor plays a role in creating chronic stress that may lead to hypertension among African-Americans: racism or, more precisely, the emotions that racism evokes among those on the receiving end of it. How many of us, no matter where we live or what our financial position, have not experienced the sting of racism? And how do we feel when we know we are being judged negatively on the basis of our skin color alone? Anger, shame, and despair are a few of the emotions that course through us every day we are forced to suffer discrimination. Many of us also feel completely powerless—powerless against the force of racism that keeps us from attaining our dreams. Thomas K., the patient you met at the beginning of this chapter, is a good example. His anger at being bypassed for promotion because of racism was compounded by the fact that he felt there was nothing he could do to change his situation.

The combination of anger and powerlessness that racism evokes may be what is doing our health the most damage. A study conducted by Cheryle Armstead of St. Louis University and Kathleen A. Lawler of the University of Tennessee proves this correlation: Armstead and Lawler showed a group of black students scenes from several movies. The scenes were divided into three categories: nonracist anger-provoking scenes; racist anger-provoking scenes; and neutral scenes. The researchers found that although blood pressure rose in everyone who viewed anger-provoking scenes, the increase was much more significant in those who viewed racist scenes. Their conclusion was that racism can have a direct effect on our blood pressure, and that if we are exposed to racism continuously, it may in fact contribute to the development of hypertension.

Stress, Coping Behavior, and Cardiovascular Disease

As mentioned earlier in this chapter, scientists have determined that it is not the *amount* of stress we face, but rather how we cope with stress that most affects our health. In the mid-1970s, two California cardiologists, Drs. Meyer Friedman and Ray Rosenman, studied the behavior of their fellow doctors and their patients. They discovered that certain behaviors were more likely to exist in people with heart disease than in others. Heart disease was more common in people they termed "Type A"; these people tended to be more demanding, ambitious, and hostile. Those with less evidence of heart disease, termed Type B, were calmer and more easygoing—although equally ambitious and successful in many cases.

In a study conducted at Duke University in North Carolina, this theory was put to a test. More than 3,000 men (most of them white)—1,500 Type As and 1,500 Type Bs—were followed to see the effect their personalities had on their health. After eight years, it was found that Type A men had significantly more atherosclerosis than Type B men. It was calculated that the increase in atherosclerosis put the Type A men at twice the risk for having a coronary thrombosis than the Type B men.

As compelling as the Type A theory is, studies relating to it have concentrated mostly on white men in white-collar jobs. The applicability of the results to African-Americans and/or blue-collar or poor people remains

TABLE 5 **Type A Personality vs. John Henryism**

Type A	John Henryism
Competitive	Struggles to "do better"
Tremendous sense of time urgency	Doesn't ask for help
Often does two things at once	Feels boxed in
Hostile	Sets high goals, but constantly feels
Low self-esteem	frustrated in achieving them
Compares self to others	
Needs to win to prove something to self and others	

unknown. While it is likely that some African-Americans are, by nature, Type A's—aggressive overachievers—racism and social injustice could lead other blacks to respond with hostility and aggressiveness that closely resemble Type A behavior.

In addition, as discussed earlier, racial discrimination also evokes a feeling of powerlessness in many African-Americans, and this perception may be another factor that predisposes blacks to developing hypertension. Dr. Sherman A. James, a researcher at the University of Michigan, developed a theory about blacks and the way we cope with stress he termed "John Henryism." John Henry, an enduring figure in African-American folklore, was a black steel worker who challenged a steam-driven machine in a battle of speed and strength. John Henry beat the machine but then died of exhaustion. His intense determination against great, if not impossible, odds remains to many a symbol of the black struggle for equality, justice, and the simple ability to get by in this world. It also helps to depict a strategy many of us have used to cope with the stress we confront in our day-to-day lives.

People who display John Henryism are likely to set very high goals and pursue them with ambition but at the same time feel trapped by forces beyond their control. When goals are not met, John Henry personalities will feel dejected and ashamed but also unwilling to give up the struggle against what they perceive—and perhaps rightly so—are impossible odds. The stress such persistent emotions places on the nervous system may indeed raise the blood pressure to hypertensive levels (Table 5).

What does all the research about stress, Type A personalities, and John Henryism mean to the average patient who comes to me with hypertension and/or heart disease? What does it mean to you? Since it is impossible to determine with any certainty what causes cardiovascular disease in a given individual, all risk factors—including stress and how you cope with it—must be taken into consideration. Although it is unlikely that you'll be able to completely change either the circumstances under which you live—racism, unfortunately, is apt to be with us for the foreseeable future—or your personality, if you know that you are repressing hostility and anger, you may be able to learn ways to express those feelings appropriately instead of simply seething in silence.

REDUCING STRESS IN EVERYDAY LIFE

One of the most effective means of reducing stress in your life is to reach out to those around you for help. Make time to sit in the kitchen and chat with your friends about your troubles and your dreams. Shoot some hoops with the guys down the street—not only will you get some exercise, but you're apt to release some tension at the same time.

Another significant stress-buster is any activity that makes you feel useful. There are literally hundreds of ways—big and small—to give of yourself to help the community. Volunteer in a literacy program. Organize some children and pick up litter on your block. Visit shut-ins in your neighborhood. Read to the sick or blind. Teach some teenagers how to paint a house. Register voters. Become a Big Brother or Big Sister.

If you are a religious person, becoming more active in your church can be a tremendously rewarding experience. It can expand your social support network, help you find a minister or priest you can trust and open up to, and get you involved in serving your community through church outreach activities. These are all easy ways to connect yourself to those around you and instill in yourself a sense of purpose. The increased self-esteem and confidence that are sure to result from this commitment will help you maintain a positive outlook on life and reduce your level of stress.

If you're interested in a more individualized approach to reducing stress, there are several options available to you—from psychotherapy to biofeedback to meditation—that can help you achieve your goal of relaxation and reduced stress. It may seem silly to have to "practice" relaxing, but for many individuals, rest and relaxation do not come easily. In fact, for many people, *trying* to relax can be a stressful activity in itself. If you relate relaxation with laziness, for instance, it's unlikely that you'll be able to help control your blood pressure by taking a nap every afternoon. The following techniques have proved helpful to many people.

Psychotherapy

Psychotherapy, treatment for emotional or mental problems through intellectual rather than medical means, is a relatively new option for many African-Americans. Until recently, very few of us felt comfortable in telling our problems to a stranger, and a great number of us simply believed that psychotherapy was useless. It can also be prohibitively expensive. In the last five to ten years, however, there has been an increase in the number of blacks who seek psychotherapy to help them cope with their problems.

There are several schools of psychological thought. Psychoanalysis and psychodynamics explore your unconscious motivations, desires, and needs. Behavioral psychology rejects the idea of unconscious motivations and instead focuses you on identifying environmental factors that stimulate you to act or react in certain ways. While psychoanalytic and psychodynamic approaches may be useful in helping patients get to the root of their problems, behavioral psychotherapists appear to have the most immediate success in getting patients to lower their blood pressures. If you think you might benefit from psychoanalysis, you may want to decide to discuss the matter with your physician and ask his or her advice in finding a reputable therapist in your area. Keep in mind that many black patients find that African-American therapists are sometimes more helpful in understanding the special stresses and strains on the black community than some white therapists. Again, it is important to discuss the matter with your physician.

Biofeedback

Biofeedback is a form of "problem-centered" therapy for hypertension. Its underlying premise is that high blood pressure can be reduced if the person suffering from it learns to control the bodily responses involved. Biofeedback was developed when studies showed that animals could control their autonomic functions such as blood pressure, by being given a reward or a punishment. Physicians adapted those findings to design ways for humans to control unconscious functions through conscious thought.

There are many biofeedback methods. One involves monitoring patients with a machine equipped with lights similar to traffic lights. A special blood pressure cuff that has a microphone that will project the sound of any changes in blood pressure is attached to the patient's arm. As blood pressure rises, the lights on the machine, as well as the sounds being emitted by the microphone, let the patient monitor the level of blood pressure. If it goes too high, for instance, the machine's lights may blink red; if pressure is normal, the light will turn yellow; if it's too low, it may blink green. The patient will learn to control his blood pressure by consciously calming down if the pressure is too high, or by thinking about stressful situations if the pressure is too low. The goal is for the patient to continue this method of blood pressure control without the need for the monitoring machine. Over time, you would learn to both recognize the normally automatic physiological changes present with hypertension and also to control them. (For more information about biofeedback, see the Resources section.)

Meditation

The word *meditation* often conjures up images of Buddhist or Hindu monks sitting cross-legged in austere rooms, chanting "ohm." While meditation is indeed an integral part of many Eastern religions, it is also an effective relaxation tool that need not have anything to do with religious practice. Meditation for relaxation requires no special training, and it can be done at any time of day and in any comfortable space. All it takes is about fifteen minutes of uninterrupted quiet.

Meditation is effective both in reducing general stress and in lowering your blood pressure. When you meditate, you quiet the sympathetic nervous system, thereby reducing the heart rate, breathing rate, and blood pressure, and causing a shift in brainwave activity that may last for hours after the meditation session. In addition to its physical benefits, meditation can help you psychologically by allowing you to focus on the cause of your stress and find ways to change how you respond to the challenges you face.

There are many good books on meditation that go into great detail about the proper sitting positions, what to expect, even what to chant. But the basic elements of meditation are very simple and can be mastered by anyone willing to set aside a few minutes a day.

BASIC MEDITATION EXERCISE

This is a simple meditation exercise that can help you relax and focus your attention away from the things that cause stress in your life. Start by sitting a few minutes—perhaps just five to ten—until the practice becomes comfortable to you.

1. Make sure you are wearing comfortable, loose, nonbinding clothing. Sweatpants or shorts and a T-shirt are ideal.
2. Find a quiet place where you will not be disturbed. Try not to sit anyplace where you might be easily distracted, such as in front of a window.
3. Sit on the floor in a comfortable position. If you can't sit on the floor, sit in a straight-backed chair.
4. Allow your hands to rest on your legs.
5. Lower your gaze so that your eyes are almost, but not quite, closed.
6. Take a deep breath and let it out slowly.
7. The easiest way to begin meditation is to count your breaths. Inhale, count one. Exhale, count two. Inhale, count three. Exhale, count four. Do this to ten and then start again with one.
8. Sit for about five minutes the first week or so (try timing yourself with a kitchen timer so that you don't have to keep track of the time). Gradually increase the time you meditate to fifteen to thirty minutes a day.

There are other relaxation techniques, such as imagery (visualizing positive changes in your life, relaxing places, or happy events) and yoga. If you'd like to explore some of the other techniques available, see the Resources section.

In the meantime, your work to lower your risk of developing hypertension and heart disease is far from over. For most people, hypertension is not caused *solely* by tension or stress. Instead, stress may act as a trigger, exacerbating or heightening other risk factors. Someone under stress who is already overweight or has a problem properly metabolizing salt, for instance, is more likely to have a chronic blood pressure problem than someone under stress without these other factors present. In the next chapter, you'll take a look at how the food you eat every day may be affecting your health.

IMPORTANT QUESTIONS AND ANSWERS ABOUT COPING WITH STRESS

Q. I've been diagnosed with hypertension, and when I get angry, my heart starts to beat faster, my palms start to sweat, and I feel agitated. Is my blood pressure higher at this point than at others? Should I take more medicine?

A. You should not take more medication. Remember, hypertension means that your blood vessels and heart are working harder *all the time*, not just when you're angry or upset. In fact, it is natural for blood pressure to rise at times of stress and then to return to a normal healthy level when the crisis is over. If you've been diagnosed with hypertension, it means that your blood pressure is elevated all the time. The medicine you've been prescribed works to keep your blood pressure at a healthy level at all times—and that involves allowing heart rate and blood pressure to rise for a short time during periods of stress.

Q. I'm under a lot of stress—I'm a single mother with two kids and two jobs. I'm wondering if the stress vitamins I see in the drugstore will help me stay healthy.

A. Unfortunately, no nonprescription medicine or formula will help you reduce the impact stress has on your body. Although your body may need more vitamins during periods of *physical* stress, such as after surgery or an injury, emotional and psychological stress are unaffected by specific vitamins, minerals, or elixirs. Eating a well-balanced diet (one without caffeine or too much sugar) and exercising will do far more for your nerves and your cardiovascular system than taking vitamins. (For more information about how vitamins and minerals work in your body, see Chapter 6.)

Q. My wife thinks I'm a little crazy, but every night after I get home from work, I spend five or ten minutes writing down everything that I have to do the next day and all the things that are bothering me. I think it helps me relax, but my wife claims that it only makes my problems seem more important than they are. Who's right?

A. More than likely, you are. A study at Pennsylvania State University showed that people were able to reduce their anxiety levels by setting aside a "worry period" every day. If they started to fret about their problems or future tasks at other times in the day, they forced themselves to postpone it until that period. The organization such a system provided gave the subjects a feeling of control that calmed them down. I'd say you are on the right track.

CHAPTER 6

Eating Right for a Healthy Heart

First, the good news. Americans today—black and white alike—appear to know more and care more about a healthy diet than ever before. Everywhere you look, from fast-food restaurants to grocery store shelves, you'll find more food that has less fat, less sodium, less sugar, and fewer harmful additives than in the past. As a result, some surveys show that the average amount of fat in the typical American diet has dropped from a high of 42 percent in 1960 to its current level of about 35 to 37 percent.

On the other hand, there's still a long way to go, especially in many African-American communities where a traditional high-salt, high-fat diet still reigns supreme. Such a diet puts us at greater risk for a host of diseases, including cardiovascular disease. This is true for two interrelated reasons. First, both salt and fat directly affect the heart and blood vessels: for most African-Americans, excess salt raises the level of fluid in the body, thus raising blood pressure and—for blacks and whites alike—excess circulating fat collects in blood and coronary vessels, causing atherosclerosis and, in many cases, heart attacks and strokes.

Second, high-salt, high-fat diets also tend to be high in calories; eating such a diet often leads to obesity. Obesity—being 20 percent over one's ideal weight—is epidemic among black Americans today, especially black women, and is itself a major risk factor for cardiovascular disease. Indeed, obese people of any race have higher rates of strokes, heart attacks, atherosclerosis, diabetes, and kidney disorders than their thinner counterparts. Needless to say, those who are significantly overweight die more often at a younger age than their thinner peers.

A balanced diet—one that provides you with the nutrients you need without overdosing you with fat, sodium, and extra calories—is crucial to your overall health and the health of your cardiovascular system. In this chapter, we'll discover just what a balanced diet really is and how best to fit the foods you need—and enjoy—into your diet every day. Special attention will be paid to the most important factors in the diet of someone striving for cardiovascular health: fat, cholesterol, sodium, potassium, and certain vitamins and minerals known as antioxidants. Then, at the end of the chapter, you'll learn the fundamentals of healthy weight loss.

THE WELL-BALANCED DIET: A PRIMER

The human body requires about forty different essential nutrients in order to carry out its functions and maintain its health. These nutrients include oxygen, water, protein, carbohydrates, fats, and a host of vitamins and minerals. The body receives oxygen from the air you breathe; without it, you could not survive for more than a few minutes. Although most of us take oxygen for granted, study after study proves that the more oxygen you supply to your body's cells—by breathing deeply and circulating more oxygen-rich blood during aerobic exercise—the better. (More about aerobic exercise in Chapter 7.)

Water, which is found in most everything we eat and drink, is another substance we tend to take for granted.

Water regulates body temperature, circulation, and excretion, and aids in digestion. It bathes virtually all of our cells in moisture. Nevertheless, few of us drink the sixty-four ounces of water our body needs every day to stay healthy.

The other thirty-eight or so essential nutrients are found in the food we eat. What we call a "balanced" diet is one that contains the appropriate amount—not too little and not too much—of those nutrients on a daily basis. In addition, a balanced diet also involves providing the right amount of calories—the energy value of food—to maintain proper body weight. A calorie represents the amount of energy the body would need to burn in order to use up that bit of food; any excess energy is stored as fat.

Most of us grew up with the idea that a balanced diet included equal amounts of four food groups: dairy, grains, meats, and fruits/vegetables. Today we know that eating right is a little more complicated than that. In fact, there are six different types of food—carbohydrates, fruits, vegetables, dairy, protein, and fats—and we need to eat each of those six foods in very different proportions because each contains different amounts of nutrients and calories.

To help you sort things out, the U.S. Department of Agriculture developed a very beneficial way of looking at our diet. Called the Pyramid Plan, it organizes food types into a triangle of different-sized boxes. Each box represents a type of food and the proportion of the daily diet it should comprise (Figure 4).

Carbohydrates form the base of the pyramid and should make up the bulk of a nutritious diet. At the much smaller tip of the triangle is fat; as you can see, fat should form a very small portion of your day's diet. In between are proteins, dairy products, and fruits and vegetables, all of which are to be eaten in varying proportions. The actual quantity of food you'll want to eat will depend on how many calories you, as an individual, burn on a daily basis, but the *proportions* of each type of food remain the same for everyone.

Let's take them one by one. *Carbohydrates* are the

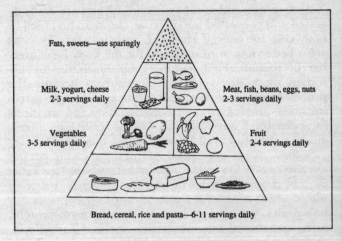

Figure 4 The Pyramid Plan

body's major source of energy; once digested, they are broken down and either immediately used as fuel (called glucose) by the cells or stored in the liver or muscles for later use (glycogen). Once the storage space is overloaded, however, any excess glucose will be stored as fat. Carbohydrates are formed by plants as a product of photosynthesis; thus all plant material, including grains, fruits, and vegetables, contain some carbohydrates.

There are three major types of carbohydrates: simple, complex, and dietary fiber. *Simple carbohydrates* are the sugars, which include glucose and fructose from fruits and vegetables, lactose from milk, and sucrose from cane or beet sugar. In their refined form, simple carbohydrates are better known as table sugar. During the refining process, carbohydrates lose much of their nutritional value but retain their calories.

Complex carbohydrates, also known as starches, are found in bread, cereals, grains, pasta, fruits, and vegetables. They are called complex carbohydrates because they consist of long chains of simple sugar molecules. Complex carbohydrates usually contain some dietary fiber as well (see Table 6).

Both simple and complex carbohydrates are easily digested and converted into glucose, the main fuel used by body cells for energy. However, complex carbohydrates are a better source of nutrition for the body for a number of reasons. First, complex carbohydrates are absorbed more slowly by the bloodstream because the process of digestion is more complicated. Simple carbohydrates—the sugars—need less digestion and are therefore absorbed more quickly by the cells; any excess glucose, therefore, will be stored more quickly as fat.

Second, foods composed of complex carbohydrates are also usually low in fat, high in dietary fiber (see Table 6), and come with a lot of nutritional extras. A slice of whole wheat bread, for instance, not only contains carbohydrates, but also packs about two grams of protein, fiber, and several other nutrients, including riboflavin, thiamine, niacin, calcium, and iron. Simple carbohydrates, on the other hand, usually come in high-calorie, high-fat packages, like cookies and cakes. If the carbohydrates you eat are complex carbohydrates, you are likely to lose, not gain, weight. If you consume too many simple carbohydrates, on the other hand, you're bound to put on pounds.

Dietary fiber, also called roughage, is the third type of carbohydrate present in whole grains, fruits, and vegetables. Fiber is not broken down by human digestive enzymes and therefore is not absorbed into the bloodstream. Although it provides no nutrients, fiber helps aid in digestion and helps keep the digestive tract clean and clear.

Dietary fiber also helps to lower blood pressure, although exactly how it does so is still poorly understood. It may be related to lowering the amount of insulin—the hormone that breaks down glucose—circulating in the blood. It might also help the body to excrete more sodium.

There are two kinds of fiber, insoluble and soluble. Insoluble fiber acts like a sponge, absorbing many times its weight in water. As it moves through the digestive tract, it pushes food along with it, then out of the body through waste elimination. Soluble fiber, on the other hand, appears to help reduce blood fat levels, thus reducing the risk of atherosclerosis. According to the American Heart Association and the USDA, the average American should consume about twenty to thirty grams of fiber every day. (See Table 6 for a list of good sources of dietary fiber.)

Fruits and Vegetables

Although occupying separate sections in the USDA's pyramid, fruits and vegetables are often combined in discussions about nutrition because they include many of the same nutrients and provide us with the same overall health benefits. Both fruits and vegetables generally are, with a few exceptions, low in fat and calories, high in fiber, and chock-full of vitamins and minerals. In fact, fruits and vegetables combine to provide about 92 percent of the vitamin C and half of the vitamin A in the nation's food supply, while contributing just 9 percent of the calories.

Most fruit is higher in sugar and calories than most vegetables. On the other hand, some vegetables contain such high levels of complex carbohydrates that they are classified as starches. These starchy vegetables include potatoes, corn, peas, and some types of beans (black, fava, kidney, lima, and soy), among others. That is not to say that these foods are not good for you: in fact, starchy vegetables are among the best sources of fiber and vitamins available. However, compared with leafy green vegetables like collard greens, kale, and spinach—which also have high fiber content—starchy vegetables are much higher in calories.

Protein

The term *protein* comes from the Greek word *protos,* which means "first and foremost." Indeed, proteins are found in every body cell, are the second most plentiful substance (after water) in the body of a normal weight person, and constitute about one-fifth of a normal adult's body weight. Protein is the major component of our muscles, organs, bones, skin, antibodies, some hor-

TABLE 6 Fiber Content of Foods

The Federal Food and Drug Administration's Center for Food Safety and Applied Nutrition recommends a range of 20 to 35 grams of dietary fiber a day.

Foods	Portion	Fiber (grams)
Bread, whole wheat	1 slice	2.7
White rice, cooked	1 cup	.8
Brown rice, cooked	1 cup	2.4
Apple, with skin	1 small	3.9
Apricots, with skin	2 medium	1.5
Kidney beans	½ cup	4.5
Peas, green	½ cup	5.2
Lima beans	½ cup	1.4
Almonds	10	1.0
Broccoli	½ cup	2.4
Lettuce	½ cup	.5

mones, and virtually all enzymes (substances that speed up the rate of biochemical actions).

Protein molecules are made up of organic compounds called amino acids. There are twenty-two amino acids; of these, the body can manufacture all but ten. These ten are called "essential amino acids" and they must be obtained from the diet. Meat, fish, egg whites, milk, and other animal products are the best sources of dietary protein. Plant material, specifically grains, legumes (certain beans and peas), and certain vegetables also contain varying amounts of protein, but no one plant source provides all of the essential amino acids in the right amount for human use.

Although animal products appear to be the best source of protein, they also are often filled with saturated fats and calories. A one-ounce slice of cheddar cheese, for instance, may contain seven grams of protein, but 71 percent of its calories come from fat. Even extra-lean hamburger, broiled well-done, derives about 52 percent of its calories from fat.

Fish, on the other hand, is an excellent source of protein, and most species contain minimal amounts of calories, fat, and cholesterol. Fish also supplies certain vitamins—particularly B vitamins—and are a good source of potassium. When choosing foods to meet your protein requirement, make sure to include fish in at least three to five meals per week.

Protein makes up nearly 25 percent of the typical African-American diet, almost twice the recommended 12 to 15 percent, which may help explain why obesity is so common. Contrary to popular belief, eating more protein than is needed *will not* add to muscle development or athletic prowess. In fact, just the opposite is true. Excess protein, like carbohydrates, is usually stored as fat.

Dairy

Although adults require just two servings—about two cups of milk or two ounces of cheese—every day, most of us neglect this aspect of our diet. Not only do milk and milk products such as cheese and yogurt provide our major source of calcium—which is essential to the health of our bones, especially as we get older—but they also are good sources of protein, carbohydrates, and vitamins and minerals.

Some of us refrain from consuming enough dairy products because we fear their naturally high calorie and fat content, others because we cannot digest them properly. In fact, as many as 70 percent of African-Americans may be lactose-intolerant: they produce abnormally small quantities of the enzyme lactase, which breaks down the milk's lactose (milk sugar) in the intestines. Many people who are lactose-intolerant, however, are able to tolerate fermented milk products, such as clabber—buttermilk traditionally used in Southern black cooking—or yogurt since some of the lactose is already broken down by the bacterial cultures in these products. In addition, many dairy companies now produce milk already treated with the enzyme lactase to aid in the digestive process.

If you are unable to consume the recommended daily portion of dairy products, you must substitute other foods rich in calcium in order to preserve your health. Later on in this chapter, you'll read more about calcium, calcium-rich foods, and the potential benefits of calcium substitutes.

Fat

Our "soul food" emphasizes fried meats and lots of fat used for seasoning and cooking. Mainstream America's most popular foods are similarly high in fat: red meat, ice cream, and fast food. Although consuming these foods on occasion is of little consequence, a regular diet rich in fat clearly has negative effects on your health.

In past centuries, fat was a survival food. Deep frying was a good preservative as well as a source of calories in a diet that otherwise might not have contained enough energy to support heavy manual labor. Today, we no longer need nearly as much extra energy since most of us live fairly sedentary lives. Although we do need to consume a little fat every day to stay healthy (the equivalent of about one tablespoon), we tend to eat too much fat simply because we think it tastes good. Fat in our foods gives it the desirable smoothness that we love. In addition, fat causes the stomach to empty more slowly, thereby giving us more "satisfaction" to the bite.

If you're like most black Americans, you need to reduce the amount and type of fat in your diet. By doing so, you'll kill at least two birds with one dietary stone. First, by reducing fat you'll automatically reduce calories, helping you lose weight if you need to or more easily maintain your weight. Second, and just as important, lowering your daily intake of fat will help you guard against the development of atherosclerosis and heart disease. Keep in mind that even if you're not overweight, you may still be consuming too much cholesterol and fat, which then circulate through the bloodstream, damaging vessels along the way.

While limiting the amount of total fat, it's important

that you keep a close watch on the kind of fat you consume as well. There are three kinds of fats—saturated, monounsaturated, and polyunsaturated—that are found in varying amounts in all foods that contain fat. Packaged foods are usually labeled by the fat that dominates in it, even though other kinds of fat may also be present.

- *Saturated fats* include animal products such as whole milk, some cheeses, butter, meat, cream, and hydrogenated vegetable shortenings. One way to recognize a saturated fat is that it is solid at room temperature. Saturated fats are the fats to avoid; they tend to raise the level of cholesterol in the blood by 5 to 10 percent.
- *Unsaturated fats,* also called polyunsaturated fats, consist of liquid vegetable oils like sunflower, corn, soybean, and sesame. These fats may actually lower the amount of cholesterol in our bodies.
- *Monounsaturated fats,* like peanut oil and olive oil, also remain liquid at room temperature. These fats do not change the amount of cholesterol or add to the amount of fat in the bloodstream.

Most fatty foods contain a combination of saturated and unsaturated fats, and all kinds of fats contain a large number of calories. For these two reasons, it's recommended that people who are eating for a healthy heart and cardiovascular system limit the amount of fat to about 30 percent of a day's total calories (400 calories or less for those dieting to lose weight) and make sure that less than 10 percent of that amount consists of saturated fats.

What Is Cholesterol?

Thanks to efforts by the American Heart Association and other health organizations, the word is out that consuming too much cholesterol is bad for our health. And in general, people are aware of the major food risks—butter, eggs, cheese, and red meat. And yet, there is still a great deal of misconception about what cholesterol is and how it affects our circulatory system.

Cholesterol is a lipid (a fatlike substance) found only in animal products like egg yolks, animal fats, cream, and cheese, to name just a few. Although cholesterol is essential for a number of vital body processes, including nerve function and cell reproduction, there is no need for anyone to consume any cholesterol at all; the body manufactures all it needs. The average American, however, consumes anywhere from 600 to 1,500 milligrams of cholesterol each day, which is from two to five times the 300-milligram limit most physicians recommend.

As you may remember from Chapter 1, there are several types of cholesterol. The two most important types in terms of cardiovascular disease are HDLs (the "good" cholesterol) and LDLs (the "bad" cholesterol). When you have more LDLs than HDLs, your body is transporting more cholesterol *into* the bloodstream, which increases your risk for atherosclerosis and heart disease. If there is more LDL in your blood, you are said to have more "bad" cholesterol, since more of this fatty substance stays in the bloodstream than is eliminated. However, it is important to note that HDL—the "good" cholesterol—is formed only in the body. You can't eat good cholesterol; *all cholesterol you eat is bad for you.*

Cholesterol is found in a wide variety of foods, and it is quite easy to consume far too much of it if you're not careful. One egg yolk, for instance, contains 250 to 275 milligrams of cholesterol; two eggs for breakfast means that you're already over your limit for the day. In addition to the well-publicized culprits like fried foods, eggs, red meat, cheese and butter, other not so obvious foods—like avocados and some shellfish, such as lobster and shrimp—are also high in cholesterol.

Vitamins and Minerals

Vitamins and minerals are substances that your body requires in certain amounts to help regulate metabolic functions within cells. They are essential to life. Without enough vitamin D, for instance, children develop rickets, a serious, degenerative bone condition. Too much sodium, at least in those people who are salt-sensitive—a majority of whom are African-American—may cause high blood pressure.

Generally speaking, only very tiny amounts of vitamins and minerals are required to carry out the body's metabolic functions. If you eat a balanced diet, you should receive all the nutrients you need from the food you eat. Contrary to popular belief, taking more vitamins and minerals than your body requires—in the form of supplements or from the diet—will not in most cases provide you with extra health benefits or make you super-strong. In fact, an overdose of some nutrients can be quite harmful.

That said, recent studies reveal that certain vitamins, particularly vitamins C, E, and beta-carotene (a precursor of vitamin A), may be especially helpful in fighting disease. These vitamins contain substances called antioxidants, which destroy certain molecules in the body called free radicals. Free radicals are known to contribute to many diseases, including heart disease. It takes oxidation by a free radical to turn cholesterol into LDL, for instance. Vitamins known to contain antioxidants appear to deactivate free radicals, thereby helping to prevent the buildup of LDL and the resulting atherosclerosis.

One study of the role of antioxidants on heart disease was reported by Drs. Joann Manson and Charles Hennekens of Harvard Medical School and Brigham and Women's Hospital in Boston. After monitoring the diet and vitamin use of 87,000 nurses for more than a decade, the investigators found that the women whose vitamin E consumption was in the upper 20 percent had a 35 percent lower risk of heart disease, even when all other factors, like smoking, blood pressure, and cholesterol, were taken into account. Those whose beta-carotene consumption was in the upper 20 percent had a 22 percent lower risk of heart disease.

Does this mean we should all take megadoses of vitamins? No—or at least not yet. The studies, although

TABLE 7 Important Vitamins and Minerals

The body needs some forty different vitamins and minerals to flourish and function properly. Many of these nutrients must come from the foods we eat. Listed below are a few of the more important nutrients, the USDA's recommended daily allowances for each, and which foods contain them in quantity.

Nutrient	RDA	Food Source
Vitamin A	800 RE	whole milk, butter, eggs, green leafy and yellow vegetables, liver, fish, apricots
Vitamin C	60 mg	citrus fruits, strawberries, tomatoes, green leafy vegetables
Vitamin D	5–10 mcg	fortified milk, fish, liver, egg yolks, butter
Vitamin E	8 mg	nuts, wheat germ, vegetable oils, whole grain cereals, olives, spinach
Calcium	1,500 mg	milk and milk products, green leafy vegetables, shellfish, citrus fruits, sardines
Potassium	no RDA (at 1,875–5,625 mg)	bananas, dried fruits, peanut butter, oranges, yogurt, dried peas, beans
Sodium	no RDA (less than 2,400 mg)	table salt, baking soda, processed foods, eggs, milk, poultry, fish, meat, breads, cereals

promising, are far from conclusive. Therefore, you should try to get your vitamins and minerals the natural way—by eating a healthful diet (Table 7).

Sodium

Sodium, a mineral found in nearly everything we eat, is directly related to hypertension in an alarming number of African-Americans. If consumed in large quantities over time, sodium may raise blood pressure to hypertensive levels, although most people who eat too much salt excrete it through urination or perspiration. As discussed in Chapter 2, however, certain people appear to be salt-sensitive; that is, their blood pressures react to salt. Salt sensitivity is believed to be genetically determined. Researchers believe that among the general population about half of all hypertensives are salt-sensitive; among African-Americans, the percentage is believed to be as high as 70 or 80 percent.

TABLE 8 Sodium Content of Common Foods

Food	Amount	Sodium (mg)
Bacon	1 slice	442
Bologna	1 slice	230
Catsup	1 tablespoon	156
Cheese (cheddar)	1 ounce	176
Corn chips	1 ounce	218
Frankfurter	1	460
Lobster (steamed)	3 ounces	326
Milk (1% fat)	1 cup	123
Pancakes	3 cakes	450
Pizza (cheese)	¼ of 12" pie	673
Sausage (pork)	1 link	1,020
Soup (canned chicken noodle)	1 cup	1,107
Soy sauce	1 tablespoon	975
Tuna	6½ ounces	519

Because no effective means have been devised to distinguish between those people who are salt-sensitive and those who aren't, most doctors recommend that we *all* decrease the amount of sodium we consume. And we consume quite a lot. Although the actual physiological need for sodium may be as low as 220 milligrams a day, most of us consume nearly twenty times that amount, or 5,000 milligrams each day. The recommended limit, set by the American Heart Association, is less than 2,400 milligrams per day.

The main source of sodium in the black American's diet is sodium chloride, commonly known as table salt. In that form, it is used as a spice and as a preservative and is found in greater or lesser amounts in nearly everything we eat. One of the first steps you should take to reduce the amount of salt you eat is to throw away the salt shaker—not just the salt you put on your food at the table, but also the salt you use to spice the food while you cook it. Although you may think you won't enjoy the taste, you'd be surprised at how quickly you'll learn to enjoy the flavor of real, unadulterated food.

The second step in your quest for salt reduction may be a bit more difficult: Avoid processed foods (including

TABLE 9 All-Purpose Spice Blend

5 tsp onion powder
2½ tsp garlic powder
2½ tsp paprika
2½ tsp powdered mustard
1¼ tsp thyme leaves
½ tsp ground white pepper
¼ tsp celery seed

Combine all ingredients and spoon into a shaker. Makes about ⅓ cup, with approximately 0.46 mg sodium per teaspoon. (Courtesy of the American Spice Trade Association.)

canned soups, fruits, and vegetables, and frozen dinners that are not specifically labeled "low-sodium"), fast-food restaurants, and snack foods. It is essential that you check food labels for sodium content—even foods that don't taste salty may be loaded with the stuff. Breakfast cereals are notoriously salty, for instance, as is American cheese and tuna fish. (See Table 8 for more information.)

You may find that reducing salt intake is difficult and that you miss the way it makes food taste. However, the longer you go without it, the less you'll miss it—and the more you'll savor the true flavors of food. To perk up the natural flavor of food, try using spices and herbs such as tarragon, pepper, basil, oregano, cumin, parsley, ginger, and the list goes on. There are hundreds of low-salt cookbooks available should you want to further experiment with herbs, wine, and other cooking methods to help spice up life-after-salt. I guarantee that within three weeks, your appetite for salt will have diminished enormously. In the meantime, several salt-substitutes are available in your supermarket, or you can sprinkle the spice blend found in Table 9, which is specially designed for those of us trying to reduce our daily intake of sodium, on your favorite meats, fish, and vegetables.

Potassium

A chemical essential for muscle contraction and other body functions, potassium also plays a role in helping

TABLE 10 Potassium Content of Food

Prune juice	1 cup	600 mg
Parsnips	1 cup, cooked	590 mg
Potatoes	1 large, w/skin	755 mg
Dried peas/beans	⅔ cup, cooked	250–450 mg
Banana	1 medium	440 mg
Milk products	1 cup	500 mg

the kidneys eliminate sodium from the body. In fact, many causes of secondary hypertension—high blood pressure caused by an identifiable agent—involve hypokalemia, or low levels of potassium. Potassium is found in high quantities in oranges and orange juice, peanut butter, dried peas and beans, yogurt, molasses, and meat (Table 10).

Is it possible to prevent hypertension by consuming more potassium? Probably not. But luckily, potassium is most often found in food low in sodium, so that when you reduce your intake of sodium, you often automatically increase your intake of potassium. Surveys show that black Americans eat more leafy greens and vegetables—substances naturally high in potassium—than the average American consumer. Once we cut down on the amount of sodium we eat, the naturally high levels of potassium in our diets may indeed have more of an impact on lowering our blood pressures. Please be aware that potassium supplements are not recommended under most circumstances, since too much potassium—hyperkalemia—can cause serious illness. Discuss whether or not you need extra potassium with your physician before taking supplements.

Calcium

Calcium is best known for its role in giving the hard structure to bones and teeth. Calcium also plays an important role in the cardiovascular system: it is needed for proper clotting of the blood and also helps to maintain blood pressure by controlling contraction of the muscles in blood vessel walls and heart tissue.

Milk, yogurt, and cheese products have high amounts of easily absorbed calcium. In fact, dairy products are the best sources of calcium. To avoid consuming too much fat, however, you should choose low-fat or skim versions of these products. For those of you who are lactose-intolerant or simply do not enjoy dairy products, other foods may provide you with enough calcium as well. Sardines (with the bones) and leafy green vegetables, such as turnip greens, collard greens, and broccoli, are particularly good sources.

Your goal should be to eat 1,000 milligrams or more of calcium each day—1,500 if you are a pregnant or post-menopausal woman. Table 11 provides a list of calcium-rich foods. If you experience gas and cramping after drinking milk, switch to a low-lactose milk or add lactase by drops or tablets to your food before having milk. If you find you are unable to meet your calcium needs through your diet, there are several different types of calcium supplements available. Generally, the least expensive and most widely available supplements are calcium carbonate and calcium lactate; both of these are absorbed by the body equally well, but may cause gassiness and/or constipation among some users. A more expensive form of calcium, called calcium gluconate, tends to have fewer side effects. Some over-the-counter antacids contain about 200 milligrams of calcium per tablet.

LOSING WEIGHT

As stated elsewhere in this text, obesity is a risk factor for all types of cardiovascular disease. Although losing weight—and keeping it off—can be very difficult for many of us, it is essential if we want to maintain our health.

Why is losing weight so difficult? Food is comfort for many people, but especially perhaps among African-Americans. Traditionally, we spend a large proportion of our income on food, and a large amount of family time

TABLE 11 Dietary Sources of Calcium

The best sources of calcium come from dairy products, but other foods contain high levels of the mineral as well.

Food	Portion	Calcium (mg)
Milk, whole or skim	8 ounces	300 ounces
Yogurt, skim with nonfat milk solids	8 ounces	452 ounces
Buttermilk	8 ounces	300 ounces
American cheese	1 ounce	195 ounces
Salmon, canned, with bones	3½ ounces	100 ounces
Shrimp	3½ ounces	63 ounces
Sardines, with bones	3½ ounces	240 ounces
Almonds	1 ounce	75 ounces
Blackstrap molasses	2 tablespoons	280 ounces
Bean curd (tofu)	3½ ounces	128 ounces
Broccoli, cooked	1 cup	160 ounces
Collards, cooked	1 cup	360 ounces
Kale, cooked	1 cup	200 ounces

together is spent eating. Given the importance of the meal as a family social gathering and the amount of money spent on food, many blacks place a special emphasis on eating.

Other causes of black obesity may be psychological. Lack of social support, stress due to violence in many black neighborhoods, lack of money, unfulfilling employment or unemployment—all of these factors may lower a person's sense of self-esteem and therefore lead him or her to the refrigerator for comfort. Domestic abuse and sexual abuse may also be factors; talk show host Oprah Winfrey has brought much attention to the problem of sexual abuse and the many repercussions it may have in the victim's later life, only one of which may be obesity.

Without question, black women suffer from obesity far more than black men. At least part of the reason for the disparity is cultural: Just think of the images of black women in the media—warm, loving, happy women gather broods of children to their ample breasts. Indeed, being overweight has been culturally accepted among many blacks—at least until recently—and even preferred by some. Who has not heard this age-old adage, "Nobody likes a bone but a dog"?

In addition, a black woman may overeat simply because she traditionally spends so much time in the kitchen. In a traditional home, the woman shops for and prepares almost all meals. She may do more than her share of snacking as she cooks, and quite often, the woman who prepared the food will eat bits left at the end of the meal rather than throw them away, thinking that any leftover food is being "wasted" if it is not eaten. These "bits" have just as many calories when heading for the trash as they do on a dinner plate. At the same time, there appears to be many physiological and perhaps genetic reasons that some of us gain weight while others do not—even while appearing to eat the same amount of food as our thinner counterparts.

For black women and men alike, access to environments supportive to weight loss may be both elusive and costly. Health-food restaurants and weight-loss centers are few and far between in many of our neighborhoods, and they are often prohibitively expensive. On the other hand, fast-food restaurants serving high-fat, high-salt meals proliferate. Dieting takes enormous willpower and effort, and it certainly doesn't help to be tempted by easy access to unhealthy, relatively inexpensive food.

Perhaps the most damaging, and luckily inaccurate, reason for black obesity is the misperception that preparing and eating healthy food is too expensive and time-consuming. In fact, a piece of fish topped with lemon and parsley takes just ten minutes to cook and costs about the same as a fast-food hamburger and fries. Changing the way you eat and the way you think of food, however, is sure to be a challenge but one you must make every effort to take on if you want to stay healthy.

Why Do We Gain Weight?

No doubt you've noticed that your neighbor Julia seems to be able to eat whatever she wants and never gain a pound, while you only have to *look* at a piece of pecan pie before fat creeps onto your tummy. Why do some people become overweight and others remain slim, even while appearing to eat the same amounts of food? It appears that genetics, individual metabolism, and a slew of other factors combine to determine a person's propensity to gain or lose weight. Like hypertension, obesity is a multifactorial disorder that goes hand-in-hand with other diseases—especially diabetes and atherosclerosis—that also run in families and that also predispose one to hypertension.

At the heart of the matter, however, is a simple formula. To lose weight, you must burn off more calories than you consume. Eating any kind of food, even those we deem most healthful, such as fruits and vegetables, can cause you to gain weight, if you eat more calories than you burn off. The number of calories needed by a specific individual to meet his or her energy needs depends on several factors, including age, weight, and level of exercise.

In addition, *what* you eat matters just as much as *how much* you eat. Indeed, not all foods are created equal: if two people eat the same weight of food in a day, but one person takes in 60 percent of her food in the form of complex carbohydrates while the other consumes her calories in the form of fat, the two will most likely end up with very different body shapes and weights.

Why? First, complex carbohydrates are used more efficiently than fat and are far less likely to be stored in adipose tissue. Experiments at the University of Massachusetts Medical School, for example, suggest that if you consume 100 excess carbohydrate calories, 23 of those calories will be used simply to process the food, and thus only 77 of them will potentially end up being stored as fat. But it appears that only 3 calories are burned in the processing and storing of 100 fat calories.

Second, and most important, a gram of fat provides more than twice the calories as a gram of carbohydrates; 9 calories as compared to 4. That's why an ounce of potato chips—processed in fat and totaling more than

160 calories—is more fattening than an ounce of baked potato, which contains about 30 calories and no fat at all.

Constructing a Healthy Eating Plan

The best way to diet is to eat relatively small portions of a wide variety of foods and expect to lose just 1 to 2 pounds a week. Fad diets that promise rapid weight loss and concentrate on eating just a few select foods are dangerous for many reasons. By concentrating solely on losing pounds and not on learning proper nutrition, you'll most likely fall back into the same kinds of bad eating habits that made you heavy in the first place. This kind of seesaw effect is both dangerous and counterproductive; rapid weight loss puts an extraordinary strain on the cardiovascular system and also changes the body's metabolic rate, forever lowering the number of calories your body needs to maintain vital functions. That's why people find it difficult to lose weight again after crash dieting.

Take another look at the Pyramid Plan. By adapting proper portion control, you can use the pyramid to develop a safe, healthy, and effective eating plan to lose weight. The adaptation of a plan recommended by the American Heart Association, shown in Table 12, replaces the often tedious struggle of calories and "dieting" by the more natural approach of portion control and food variety.

Carefully watching what you eat—and reducing the amount of familiar but fatty foods from your diet—may feel like a punishment, especially at first. With time, however, you may be surprised at how much you enjoy the taste of delicious, healthy food. Moreover, as the pounds drop away, you just may discover that you have more energy than you ever dreamed you had. In fact, even before actual weight is lost, your new commitment to a healthy lifestyle may prompt you to add another important component to any cardiovascular fitness plan: exercise. In the next chapter, you'll learn the principles of safe, effec-

TABLE 12 Your Daily Food Plan for Healthy Weight Loss

The following portions of protein, carbohydrates, fruits, vegetables, breads, dairy products, and fat will provide you with about 1,300 calories per day. Depending on your age and weight, this may translate into a healthy weight loss of 1 to 2 pounds a week; if you weigh more than, say 150 to 160 pounds, you may want to increase the amount of food prescribed here as well as increase your exercise level. Before beginning any eating or exercise plan, please consult with your physician.

- *4 servings of bread/starches,* each consisting of no more than 80 calories (bread, English muffins, pasta, cereal, potatoes, rice, popcorn)

- *4 to 6 ounces of protein* (chicken, turkey, fish, lean beef, veal, pork, lamb, lentils, dried peas, sprouts and grains, nuts, egg whites as desired; but only two to three whole eggs per week)

- *3 ½-cup servings (or more) of fresh vegetables*

- *3 servings of medium-sized fruit*

- *2 8-ounce servings of low-fat milk, yogurt, or cottage cheese;* this includes hard cheeses, but no more than four 1-ounce servings per week

- no more than *2 tablespoons of fats*

By following this plan, you should be able to lose weight easily and without feeling hungry.

tive activity and all about what it can do for your heart and blood pressure.

IMPORTANT QUESTIONS AND ANSWERS ABOUT EATING RIGHT FOR A HEALTHY HEART

Q. I've changed from eating butter to eating margarine. Is margarine any less fattening?

A. No. Butter and margarine each contain equal amounts of calories. However, margarine contains less saturated fat, which means less cholesterol to clog your arteries. Therefore, margarine is a better choice in terms of preventing heart disease, but it should be eaten sparingly if weight loss is also an issue.

Q. I'm supposed to be cutting down on sodium because of my high blood pressure. Is garlic salt and/or sea salt okay to use?

A. I'm afraid not. About the same amount of sodium is found in flavored salts as in regular table salt. A much better choice for you are flavored *peppers*, such as lemon pepper, or other spices. Be sure to check the label on all products you purchase for the amount of sodium they contain.

Q. I love to eat fish and hear that it's a good source of protein and pretty low in fat. Am I right?

A. As long as you don't cook your fish in fat or load it with heavy cream sauces or dressings (like tartar sauce), you've made an excellent choice for your heart and for any weight loss efforts you've embarked upon. Not only does fish tend to have less fat than meat, but the fat in fish is highly polyunsaturated, which means that it does not raise blood cholesterol levels. Moreover, fish fat contains a special group of polyunsaturated fatty acids known as omega-3s, which have been shown to protect against heart disease by reducing the tendency of the blood to clot. As you may remember from Chapter 2, blood clots that travel to coronary arteries are a leading cause of heart attacks. Omega-3s also lower triglyceride levels, another type of fat implicated in cardiovascular disease. Fish especially high in omega-3s include salmon, mackerel, herring, sardines, tuna, and anchovies.

CHAPTER 7

Exercising Your Way to Cardiovascular Fitness

"The body of research is now of sufficient strength to identify a sedentary life-style as a risk factor comparable to high blood pressure, high blood cholesterol, and cigarette smoke in the development of heart disease," announced Dr. Edward S. Cooper, president of the American Heart Association, on September 1, 1992. By making that statement, Dr. Cooper confirmed what doctors and their exercising patients have been saying for years: Whether you're black or white, young or old, male or female, exercise is good for you and good for your heart.

It is true that for most modern African-Americans, especially those who live in urban areas, getting exercise doesn't come naturally. We tend not to have the time required to exercise and/or lack the access to health facilities and the knowledge to use them. Yet, less than a century ago more than half of all Americans and even a higher percentage of African-Americans worked in jobs—agriculture, construction, etc.—that met their daily exercise needs. When our grandparents were growing up, for instance, no one joined a health club or took up jogging and there were no more fat people then than there are now; in fact, there were far fewer. Instead, they were getting all the exercise they needed—and more—in the cotton fields, construction sites, and coal mines. Today, however, fewer than 2 percent of the population have jobs that involve any kind of cardiovascular effort.

Nevertheless, it is vital that you make exercise a part of your life, especially if you have risk factors for hypertension and heart disease and—this may surprise you—even if you've had a heart attack. Mary E., a fifty-eight-year-old patient of mine who is recovering from a heart attack, was quite concerned when I suggested that she start an exercise program. She remembered that her grandfather, who'd had hypertension and at least two heart attacks, was told to stay as inactive as possible lest he "burst something" while performing even the mildest physical task.

Indeed, at one time, most people with hypertension and/or heart disease were told not to exert themselves for fear of provoking a heart attack or stroke. More and more, however, exercise conditioning is not only strongly recommended as a preventive measure, but is frequently used as a rehabilitative method in treating heart attack patients.

That said, it is extremely important that you discuss an exercise plan with your physician *before* you start to exercise. This is especially true if you've already been diagnosed with high blood pressure or heart disease or if you've already suffered a heart attack. Exercise does require your heart and blood vessels to work harder, and if they are already damaged by atherosclerosis, the extra stress could provoke a heart attack or stroke. (See below for more information on the importance of a pre-exercise stress test.)

The Benefits of Exercise

Your heart, your blood vessels, and virtually every system in your body will physiologically thank you when you add exercise to your everyday life. You're likely to find that you digest food more rapidly and easily, you'll be less likely to become constipated, you'll feel fewer aches and pains, and you'll have more energy.

Most important in the context of this book, exercise helps to prevent and reduce both high blood pressure and coronary heart disease. When you exercise, the arterioles (the smallest blood vessels) dilate or open up, which lessens their resistance to blood flow. Exercise also lowers blood pressure by decreasing sympathetic nervous system activity, thereby reducing sodium retention.

Because your muscles need more oxygen when they're at work, the heart must pump harder to get extra oxygen-rich blood to them. Normally, the heart pumps about six quarts of blood a minute in an adult, but when the body is exercising, blood volume to and from the heart rises to about twenty-five quarts per minute. This extra work strengthens the heart muscle; the stronger it is, the less hard it has to work to meet the body's need for oxygen. Exercise also helps improve the health of the entire circulatory system because it distributes blood more evenly to all the blood vessels throughout the body.

In addition, a number of studies have found that regular, vigorous exercise can both lower total blood cholesterol and increase the ratio of HDLs to LDLs. After following 500 healthy middle-aged women for three years, for instance, researchers at the University of Pittsburgh found that women who burned just 300 calories more per week than they did at the start of the study were able to maintain healthy levels of HDLs. As you know, this reduces the risk for atherosclerosis, a leading risk factor for heart attacks and strokes.

The good news for the thousands of African-American women who are struggling with obesity is that aerobic exercise is one of the best and safest ways to step up weight loss efforts. Aerobic exercise both burns calories and speeds up metabolism—the rate at which your body burns food, even when the body is at rest. About 3,500 calories comprise 1 pound of body fat; you can lose that pound by walking for ten hours (at about four miles per hour) or cross-country skiing for about six hours.

Perhaps just as important as the effects of exercise on the cardiovascular system and metabolism is the way it makes you feel about yourself and the world in general. It may sound like an impossible dream, but exercise has psychological as well as physical benefits. Think of it this way: Brain tissue is fed by thousands of tiny capillaries, so the more blood coursing through them to feed the brain, the more mentally alert and emotionally satisfied you'll feel. In addition, certain body chemicals called endorphins, known to dull pain and produce a mild euphoria, are released during vigorous exercise. Smokers find it easier to quit when they're exercising, therapists frequently prescribe exercise to their depressed patients, and dieters who also exercise claim to feel less hungry and more self-confident about meeting their weight-loss goals than they did when they were sedentary.

Designing an Exercise Program

Your first step in developing an exercise program is to consult with your physician, especially if you're overweight, over forty, have been diagnosed with heart disease or hypertension, or have any other risk factors for cardiovascular disease, including cigarette smoking, high cholesterol levels, or diabetes. Your doctor may recommend that you take a stress test, which assesses how your heart and blood vessels are functioning with exercise. As you may remember from Chapter 3, a stress test involves nothing more than having your heart rate measured by EKG (electrocardiogram) and your blood pressure monitored by a technician while you walk or jog on a treadmill or ride a stationary bicycle.

One of the most important benefits of the stress test is that it helps diagnose heart and vessel disease through changes in the EKG tracings. If your coronary arteries are severely blocked, for instance, it will most likely be revealed on an EKG. A stress test will also help determine the amount of exercise your heart and muscles can handle without any adverse effects. Both the length of time you are able to exercise and the intensity of activity you are able to endure without becoming exhausted will help your doctor determine a safe exercise routine for you.

After you receive the results of your stress test, you and your doctor can plan your exercise program. In essence, there are two basic types of exercise: aerobic (or isotonic) and anaerobic (or isometric). The purpose of aerobic exercise is to improve cardiovascular health by forcing the body to deliver ever larger amounts of oxygen to working muscles. In fact, the word *aerobic* is derived from a Greek word meaning "air." Anaerobic exercise (exercise "without air"), on the other hand, attempts to strengthen individual muscles, which draw on their own sources of energy and do not require the body to increase its supply of oxygen. Also known as muscle conditioning or weight training, anaerobic exercise tries to build muscle mass while keeping the body strong and flexible.

Please note that anaerobic exercise is *not* recommended for someone with uncontrolled high blood pressure or heart disease. The tensing of the muscles in the arms and legs causes a restriction of the blood vessels and a reduction in the flow of blood and can lead to severe hypertension. If atherosclerosis or other vessel damage already exists in the heart, brain, or blood vessels, such exercise could cause strokes or heart attacks. However, if your blood pressure is normal or even borderline, weight training may be perfectly appropriate for you. Ask your physician for advice.

In general, then, people wanting to improve cardiovascular health should concentrate on aerobic exercise, such as walking, jogging, cycling, singles tennis, skiing, rowing, even ice skating or rollerskating. Any of these activities, done regularly, will boost your heart rate and provide your body with all the benefits of exercise described above.

In order for aerobic exercise to have a healthy effect on the cardiovascular system, however, it must be of a sufficient intensity and frequency. You should exercise at a level of intensity called your target heart rate, or the rate at which your heart must work to provide health benefits to the cardiovascular system. At this rate, you will burn about 300 calories in 30 minutes.

Target heart rates are calculated by using a simple formula. Your target heart rate is between 60 and 80 percent of your maximum heart rate; your maximum heart rate is calculated by subtracting your age from 220. For the average fifty-year-old, then, your maximum heart rate would be 220 − 50, or 170. Your target heart range should be from 102 to 136 beats per minute, which is 60 to 80 percent of your maximum heart rate. For the average target heart rates for the average adult thirty years and older see Table 13.

You can determine whether or not you are within your target zone by taking your pulse immediately after exercise. To take your pulse, place two fingers (not your thumb, it is also a pulse point and can disturb the accuracy of your reading) on your wrist or on your neck just under your chin and to one side of your throat. Count the beats for 10 seconds, then multiply that number by 6. If your pulse rate is below the target range, you should increase either the intensity or the length of your workout. If your pulse is above your target rate, slow down.

In addition to being aerobic and intense, exercise must be performed on a regular basis. For cardiovascular benefits to be achieved, exercise should be done about three times a week, for at least thirty minutes, preferably at your target heart rate. Keep in mind that this is a goal to strive for; if you're not in shape or if you've already been diagnosed with hypertension or heart disease, it will take some time for you to be able to exercise at this level.

The Exercise Session

Getting enough exercise doesn't require joining an expensive health spa or buying expensive equipment. One of my patients, a thirty-eight-year-old mother of two small children named Phoebe W., decided to get her exercise the old-fashioned way: she walked it. Putting the two children (two years and nine months old) in a double stroller, Phoebe walked around the neighborhood park at a good clip, averaging about two miles in a thirty-minute period. She planned the excursion to take place during the two-year-old's nap time so that she wouldn't be fussy and the nine-month-old baby simply loved being outside. Within six months of regular walking and watching her food intake, Phoebe managed to lose almost fifteen pounds and her blood pressure had fallen several

TABLE 13 Training Heart Rates by Age

Age	60%	80%
30	111	148
40	108	144
45	105	140
50	102	136
55	99	132
60	96	128
65	93	124

points—and it didn't cost her a dime or inconvenience her in any way.

As Phoebe's case proves, walking is an excellent form of aerobic exercise. In fact, the American Medical Association has pointed out that a walk of just one mile a day at a moderate pace is a simple and pleasant way to lose weight and give your heart a decent workout. After a year of walking a mile every day, you will have lost about 36 pounds and probably incorporated exercise into your life for good.

But walking is just one of dozens of equally effective aerobic exercises, and you should choose the one that interests you the most. Regardless of the type you choose, every workout session should contain three elements: (1) a warm-up; (2) an exercise phase (either cardiovascular or muscle conditioning or both); and (3) a cool-down. Ideally, the entire session should last about forty-five to sixty minutes.

1. A ten- to fifteen minute *warm-up* is essential for your muscles. Warming up prepares you for exercise by gradually increasing your heart rate, blood flow, and muscle action. Contrary to popular belief, however, a good warm-up does not begin with stretching; stretching cold muscles can injure them. Instead, you should jog in place for a minute or two before you start to stretch. Once you feel warm, carefully begin stretching major muscle groups, including your legs, upper arms and shoul-

ders, upper back, and neck. In performing these exercises, hold each position for thirty seconds and *do not bounce*. The average stretching session should last about ten minutes.

2. The *aerobic phase* of the exercise should last approximately twenty to thirty minutes at your target heart rate. However, beginners who are out of shape may have trouble sustaining intense exercise for that long. Many experts suggest reducing this phase of the workout session to about five to ten minutes for a few weeks until your heart and muscles have gained some capacity and strength. If you decide to combine aerobics with weight training at the same time, it may be best to shorten your aerobic routine to perhaps twenty minutes.

3. If you decide you'd like to strengthen your muscles as well as work your cardiovascular system—and if you've received permission from your physician—a *weight-training* and muscle-conditioning routine could either come after an aerobic workout or be performed on a separate day after an appropriate warm-up. A weight-training routine should involve about thirty minutes of slow—but constant—stress on different muscles of the body using free weights or strength-training equipment such as Nautilus or Kaiser. Your exact exercise routine should be formulated with an exercise specialist in a gym or at the YWCA, but generally speaking, it consists of about a dozen exercises: six for the upper body and six for the lower body.

No matter what type of exercise program you choose, it is important that if you feel any of the following symptoms while exercising, *stop exercising immediately and consult your physician*. What you are feeling could be signs of cardiovascular stress, such as a heart attack or a stroke:

- Dizziness
- Headache
- Nausea

- Chest discomfort, including pain, tightness, heaviness, or breathlessness
- Any discomfort or numbness in the jaw, neck, or arm

4. The third phase of your workout session is called the *cool-down,* during which you gradually reduce the level of intensity. If you jog, for instance, don't suddenly stop and sit down. Instead, walk a block or two at a somewhat slower pace. Then stretch gently for about five to ten minutes. Cooling down will both help you avoid muscle stiffness and reduce the chances of an abrupt drop in blood pressure that can occur when exercise comes to a sudden halt.

You should perform your chosen aerobic exercise at least three times a week for a minimum of twenty minutes a session. You should also set a target pulse rate during exercise, which would be between 60 and 80 percent of your maximum heart rate. (See Table 13 on page 139 to figure your maximum and target heart rates.)

Sticking With It

You know in your heart that your exercise program should last forever and that regular exercise must become a part of your daily life if lasting health benefits are to be derived. But you've seen others fail in their same, very good intentions. Perhaps you've failed before, too.

Here are a few simple hints that will help you incorporate exercise into your daily routine for the rest of your life:

1. Start slowly. Don't overdo your exercising in the first few days. If you do, you are likely to become sore and not want to continue with your workout plan. Indeed, the best way to stick to exercising is to start small and build gradually.

2. Vary the type of exercise you do. Walk one day, bike the next, play volleyball with friends on Friday, garden on Sunday. By varying your routine, you're more likely to keep it going.

3. Find some company. For most of us, there comes a time when our motivation sags and we lose interest in exercising on a regular basis. When this happens—preferably *before* this happens—enlist a friend or loved one to join you in your quest for cardiovascular health. Often, a little competition and companionship go a long way. Many communities have organized groups that walk together in parks or malls. The National Black Women's Health Project, for instance, started a "Walking for Wellness" program that will help you organize walking groups at your workplace or in your neighborhood, church, or school. The program includes a plan for walking twenty to thirty minutes three times a week complete with imaginary walking tour tapes of Boston's Black Heritage Trail, the island of Jamaica, and Africa's Mount Kilimanjaro, among others. (For more information call the National Black Women's Health Project, 1-800-ASK-BWHP.)

4. Expand your definition of exercise. A recent study at the USDA Human Nutrition Research Center on Aging at Tufts University showed that nonathletes who merely moved around a lot in their daily lives had less body fat than those who were more sedentary. Indeed, simply being more *active* every day will do a lot to improve your overall health. Instead of taking the elevator, walk up three or four flights of stairs. Look at your household and gardening chores as great chances to stretch, lift, and bend your body instead of mere drudgery. Most important of all, put away the keys to your car and use your feet instead.

5. Choose activities you enjoy. Consider this: If you exercise for forty-five minutes three times a week for a year, you'll be spending 117 hours—the equivalent of about three full forty-hour work weeks—sweating and striving at one activity or an-

other. The likelihood that you'll stick with such a routine depends to a large degree on enjoying what you're doing every time. Finding an activity that excites or motivates you will help strengthen your resolve.

6. **Set realistic goals.** How many of us have vowed to transform ourselves into Whitney Houston or Carl Weathers by logging in two hours every day at the gym? And how many of us, after missing just one session, have declared ourselves failures and have given up completely? After failing to meet an unrealistic goal, or straining our muscles trying to do so, we often become so frustrated we decide not to exercise at all. To avoid this self-defeating trap, set goals you know you can meet, or perhaps ones just slightly out of reach. Achieving them will give you a sense of pride and self-confidence that is sure to keep you motivated.

7. **Seek convenience.** Eliminate as many excuses as possible for not exercising. If you join a health club that means driving for a half hour or riding two subways to get there, you're setting yourself up to fail. Scheduling times to exercise—and treating your exercise times as if they were business appointments—is often the only way to incorporate aerobic activity into your lifestyle.

The previous four chapters of this book have concentrated on ways to prevent developing hypertension and heart disease. Despite your best efforts, however, these nondrug therapies may not be enough to prevent high blood pressure or atherosclerosis from affecting you. If so, don't despair. In the last thirty years or so, medical science has developed several medications that will help you reduce hypertension, high cholesterol, and other cardiovascular disease. Surgical techniques to repair damaged heart tissue are more successful than ever in preventing heart attacks and strokes from occurring and in lessening their lethal effects. In Chapter 8, you'll learn about medical therapies and how they might apply to you.

IMPORTANT QUESTIONS AND ANSWERS
ABOUT EXERCISING YOUR WAY TO
CARDIOVASCULAR FITNESS

Q. I had a mild heart attack last year. I feel okay now, and my doctor wants me to start exercising, mainly to lose weight. But I'm afraid. Won't exercising put me at greater risk for another heart attack?

A. On the contrary. Studies have shown that exercising after a heart attack actually *reduces* your risk of having another one. Once you've had a stress test (see above), you and your doctor—and perhaps an exercise therapist familiar with the needs of heart disease patients—should work out a safe exercise plan for you, especially if you are taking antihypertensive drugs.

Q. I've been working out for several months. I jog three times a week for about thirty minutes each time and every other day I do some weight training in the Nautilus room at the Y. I started to exercise to lose weight—which I did—but now I see by the scale that I've gained about three pounds. I'm not eating any more than usual, so what's going on?

A. Muscle tissue is denser than fat and hence weighs more. By weight training, you are adding muscle bulk to your body even while losing fat. Although you may have netted a few pounds, you probably look thinner and firmer than before you started your exercise program, and your heart and blood vessels are no doubt much healthier.

Q. My boyfriend loves to jog, but I hate it and it hurts my knees. I say walking will burn as many calories as running, but he says jogging is better. Who's right?

A. You are, if you walk fast enough. If you can walk your mile in about fifteen minutes, you will derive just about the same cardiovascular benefits and burn around the same amount of calories as jogging a mile in a shorter amount of time.

Part III

Understanding Medical and Surgical Treatment

CHAPTER 8

Understanding Cardiovascular Drugs and Heart Surgery

Millions of Americans, black and white, are diagnosed with hypertension and/or coronary heart disease every year. As a first line of treatment, physicians usually recommend eliminating those lifestyle factors, such as smoking and obesity, that may be causing or exacerbating the condition—the risk factors you've been reading about in the previous four chapters.

Some patients, and perhaps you're one of them, require treatment with drugs and/or surgery to prevent cardiovascular disease from progressing to a medical crisis point, such as a heart attack or stroke. Perhaps you've found it impossible to lose those 20 pounds or reduce the cholesterol circulating in your bloodstream. Or perhaps your doctor feels that your blood pressure or the condition of your coronary arteries requires immediate therapy.

What determines when drug or surgical therapy is necessary in cases of hypertension and/or cardiovascular disease varies considerably from patient to patient. Before recommending any kind of treatment, your doctor will factor in your age, general health, diet, exercise habits, and other personal data.

A common question among my patients is: If drugs or surgery is available to "fix me up," why bother trying to prevent or treat cardiovascular disease by changing my lifestyle? First off, surgery of any type is stressful to the body, may be expensive, and involves certain medical risks. In addition, unless the underlying problem—specifically atherosclerosis caused by circulating cholesterol and fat—is also treated, surgery will provide only temporary relief.

Although blood pressure and cardiac drugs are quite effective and very commonly prescribed, they are not without drawbacks. Because treatment of cardiovascular disease is usually a lifelong proposition, most patients who rely on medication must take one or more pills each day, every day, for the rest of their lives. For many African-Americans, the cost of such treatment and the follow-up care they require is prohibitive, especially since many of us have no health insurance and/or access to quality health care facilities.

Furthermore, many cardiovascular drugs may produce unpleasant side effects—including lethargy, weakness, dizziness, impotence, and depression—that are often far worse than any symptoms of disease the average cardiovascular patient experiences without taking medication. Although most side effects diminish with time or can be alleviated by changing medications, they remain a fact of life for many cardiovascular patients.

For these reasons, concentrating on eliminating health risks—controlling substance abuse, reducing stress, losing weight, eating right, and exercising—is often a better choice than drug treatment for many patients, especially those of us who have only mild cases of diagnosed hypertension or coronary heart disease.

However, and this is a *big* however, you must keep in mind that, although you may have never *felt* ill in the past, your high blood pressure and/or atherosclerosis may be causing severe damage to your cardiovascular system—damage that might end up destroying a part of your brain or heart or costing you your life. If your doctor decides that drugs or surgery are necessary to help you, listen to his or her advice and then learn as much as you can about the therapy prescribed and the alternatives available to you. That way, you'll not only be better prepared for any side effects you may face, you'll also be in a position to be partner with your doctor in the decision-making process.

DRUGS FOR THE HEART AND CIRCULATION

The aim of cardiovascular drug therapy is to lower blood pressure to normal levels and/or reduce atherosclerosis and to do so with minimal side effects. As our knowledge of the underlying causes of hypertension and heart disease grows, so too does our success rate in treating these conditions with drugs.

In choosing which drug therapy is appropriate for you, your doctor will take into consideration a number of factors: the possible side effects of the drugs, how well you respond to taking the drugs, if more than one drug is needed, and other conditions or disorders you might have along with your heart and/or vessel disease.

A thorough discussion of cardiovascular drugs goes far beyond the scope of this chapter. It's up to you to consult with your physician. This part of this book will give you a general overview of both the benefits and the side effects of the major cardiovascular drugs so that you can discuss options with your physician. The major cardiovascular drug groups are listed in alphabetical order below. Included in each entry is a description of how the drugs work, what special considerations should be noted, their possible side effects, and their generic and trade names. Please note that this is an extremely abbreviated listing; no doubt you will want more information about the drug or drugs your doctor prescribes for you.

The type of drug your doctor recommends to you will depend on your symptoms and underlying condition. *An-*

tianginal drugs are prescribed to relieve chest pain caused by the lack of adequate blood supply to the heart. They do so by either improving the blood supply to the heart muscle or reducing the workload on the heart. They include *beta blockers, calcium channel blockers,* and *nitrates.*

Antihypertensive drugs are prescribed to lower blood pressure in any of several different ways. Often, more than one type of antihypertensive drug is necessary to reduce blood pressure. *ACE inhibitors, beta blockers, calcium channel blockers, diuretics, nitrates, sympatholytics,* and *vasodilators* are the groups of drugs prescribed to treat hypertension.

Anticlotting agents are used to reduce the ability of the blood to stick together and form emboli or thrombi— blood clots that clog a vital artery to the heart or brain. They include *anticoagulants, antiplatelets,* and *thrombolytics.*

Antihyperlipidemia drugs, or *lipid-lowering drugs,* are used to lower the amount of lipids (fats, cholesterol, and triglycerides) circulating in the blood.

ALPHABETICAL DIRECTORY OF CARDIOVASCULAR DRUG GROUPS

ACE Inhibitors act to prevent production of a hormone, angiotensin II, that constricts blood vessels (ACE stands for angiotensin-converting enzyme). In addition to dilating blood vessels, ACE inhibitors may also work to prevent the abnormal rise in hormones associated with hypertension and heart disease, including aldosterone, which acts on the kidneys to retain salt and water.

Special considerations: ACE inhibitors tend to be more expensive than some other cardiovascular drugs and tend to be less effective in African-Americans than whites when used alone. However, they are often effective for some black patients when paired with a diuretic (see below). They are especially useful for hypertensive diabetics and those with atherosclerosis, because ACE inhibitors rarely raise glucose or blood lipid levels as do many other medications.

Possible side effects: Dizziness or weakness, loss of appetite and/or nausea, a hacking cough, and swelling.

Generic and trade names: Captopril (Capoten); enalapril (Vasotec); lisinopril (Prinivil, Zestril).

Anticoagulants inhibit the ability of the blood to clot and prevent clots from forming or growing in blood vessels. These agents are especially useful in preventing heart attacks or strokes, since they prevent blood clots from forming around damaged tissue.

Special considerations: Anticoagulants interact with many other kinds of drugs, including aspirin (an antiplatelet drug, see below), oral contraceptives, seizure medication, and laxatives. In addition, Vitamin K tends to react with anticoagulants, and patients who eat large amounts of leafy vegetables high in vitamin K—such as kale—put themselves at increased risk of complications. (For more information about vitamin K and anticoagulants, consult your physician.) If you are pregnant or have impaired kidney or liver function, anticoagulants may not be right for you.

Possible side effects: Excessive bleeding or bruising from minor injuries and nausea and/or vomiting.

Generic and trade names: Warfarin (Coumadin, Panwarfarin).

Antiplatelets, like anticoagulants, work to keep blood from abnormally clotting. They act on a type of blood cell known as platelets by making them less sticky and thus less likely to clump together and clot. Antiplatelets are prescribed to prevent heart attacks and strokes in patients with atherosclerosis.

Special considerations: The most common antiplatelet drug regimen is low doses of aspirin taken every day. Antiplatelets also reduce the severity and frequency of angina. They should be taken with caution by patients with digestive system problems (such as ulcers), bleeding disorders, or who are pregnant or breastfeeding.

Possible side effects: Nausea or indigestion.

Generic and trade names: Acetylsalicylic acid or aspirin

(Alka-Seltzer, Anacin, Bayer, Bufferin, Ecotrin), dipyridamole (Persantine).

Beta Blockers work by blocking the action of the beta receptors in the heart, blood vessels, and other parts of the body. This stops the action of neurotransmitters that have been released by the sympathetic nervous system and thus decreases cardiac output. Beta blockers also block the production of renin—the enzyme responsible for stimulating the kidney to retain salt and water—thereby reducing some of the workload on the heart.

Special considerations: For reasons that are not yet fully understood, African-Americans do not seem to respond to some types of beta blockers as well as whites. However, when combined with a diuretic, there appears to be little difference in the way blacks and whites respond to the drugs. Beta blockers are not recommended for people with asthma (they tend to cause spasms in the bronchial tubes).

Possible side effects: Weakness, lethargy, nausea, nightmares, depression, and impotence.

Generic and trade names: Acebutolol (Sectral), atenolol (Tenormin), metoprolol (Lopressor), nadolol (Corgard), propranolol (Inderal).

Calcium Channel Blockers work to relax the muscles in vessel walls by lessening the availability of calcium—a mineral that affects the rate at which muscles contract—to the cells in the arterial walls. These drugs also cause the coronary arteries to dilate, thereby increasing the blood supply to the heart, and are thus often used to treat angina.

Special considerations: Calcium channel blockers lower blood pressure in the majority of patients who take them; however, they tend to be expensive and probably should be prescribed only when other less expensive drugs have failed.

Possible side effects: Dizziness, headache, constipation, lethargy, nausea, and swelling.

Generic and trade names: Diltiazem (Cardizem), nicardipine (Cardene), nifedipine (Procardia, Procardia XL), nimodipine (Nimotop), verapamil (Calan, Isoptin, Verelan).

Diuretics, commonly referred to as water pills, reduce the volume of the body's blood and fluids—and hence the blood pressure—by increasing the kidney's excretion of sodium and water. Treatment with diuretics causes a significant reduction in a patient's fluid volume; this lower volume lessens both heart workload and pressure on the vessel walls.

Special considerations: Diuretics remain a very effective—and the least expensive—drug to reduce hypertension, especially among African-Americans. In addition, diuretics are the only antihypertensive drugs proven—to date—to decrease the number of strokes and heart failure among patients who take them.

Today, there are three types of diuretics. The most commonly prescribed are the *thiazides,* which block the reabsorption of sodium and chloride back into the bloodstream. *Loop diuretics* are stronger drugs, usually reserved for patients with damaged kidneys. Loop diuretics, so named because they work in the part of the kidney known as the Loop of Henle, are quite potent; in fact they eliminate about 15 percent more salt from the kidneys than do the thiazides. The third type of diuretic includes the *potassium-sparing agents.* This class of drugs was developed when physicians discovered that, along with sodium, diuretics eliminated another essential mineral, potassium. Potassium is essential for proper muscle function, and that includes heart action. When potassium loss does occur, patients experience a number of dangerous side effects, including irregular heartbeat, muscle weakness, and often, glucose intolerance, which may trigger or exacerbate diabetes mellitus. Potassium-sparing diuretics work in the exchange sites of the kidneys to increase sodium excretion while maintaining potassium levels. They are usually paired with another diuretic to compensate for the potential loss of potassium.

Possible side effects: Lethargy, cramps, rash, and impotence.

Generic and trade names: Chlorthalione (Hygroton), tri-amterene/hydrochlorothiazide (Maxzide), metolazone (Diulo, Mykrox, Zaroxolyn), bumetanide (Bumex), furosemide (Lasix), amiloride (Midamor), spironolactone (Aldactone).

Lipid-Lowering Drugs lower the amount of lipids, or fats, circulating in the blood, thereby reducing or preventing atherosclerosis. There are two main types of lipid-lowering drugs—those that act on the liver by blocking the conversion of fatty acids to lipids; and those that act to reduce the absorption of bile salts (substances containing large amounts of cholesterol that are secreted from the liver into the intestine) into the blood. Different drugs affect different parts of the patient's "total lipid profile," including high-density lipoprotein (HDL), low-density lipoprotein (LDL), and triglycerides.

Special considerations: Drugs used to lower cholesterol are prescribed *only* in combination with dietary restrictions to lower the intake of fat and cholesterol. If a person on drug therapy for high blood cholesterol continues to eat a high-fat, high-cholesterol diet, the effects of the medication may be completely undermined.

Possible side effects: Constipation, bloating, nausea, headaches, diarrhea, dizziness, rapid heartbeat, insomnia.

Generic and trade names: Cholestryramine (Questran, Questran Light), colestipol (Colestid), gemfibrozil (Lopid), lovastatin (Mevacor), nicotinic acid or niacin (NiaBid, Niacels, Nicolar), probucol (Lorelco).

Nitrates, the oldest and most frequently used coronary artery medication, are potent vein and artery dilators used to treat angina pectoris and, occasionally, congestive heart failure. Nitrates relax the muscles of the blood vessels so that they dilate, thereby improving blood flow through the heart.

Special considerations: Some of these drugs interact with antihypertensive medication to lower blood pressure.

Possible side effects: Headaches, flushing, dizziness, and fainting.

Generic and trade names: Nitroglycerin (Deponit NTG, Minitran, Nitro-Bid, Nitrogard, Nitroglyn, Nitrol, Nitrolingual, Nitrong, Nitrostat, Transderm-Nitro, Tridil), isosorbide dinitrate (Dilatrate-SR, Iso-Bid, Isordil, Sorbitrate, Sorbitrate SA).

Sympatholytics, which include alpha-adrenergic drugs, work through the sympathetic nervous system to prevent the constriction of blood vessels that causes blood pressure to rise. By doing so, they widen the blood vessels in many parts of the body. There are five different types of sympatholytics, each of which works on a different part of the body. *Central-acting drugs* lower blood pressure by stimulating certain nerve receptors, located in the brain itself, which act to reduce heart rate and lower the resistance of the blood vessels. *Peripheral inhibitors* interfere with the release of norepinephrine from sympathetic nerve endings. Without norepinephrine, vessel walls will not contract and blood pressure will not rise. *Alpha blockers* are designed to lower blood pressure by dilating the arteries and arterioles. Alpha blockers often raise the level of HDLs (the "good cholesterol") while lowering total lipid levels, which is why they are especially useful to patients who suffer from both hypertension and coronary heart disease. *Beta blockers,* described above, are also considered sympatholytics.

Special considerations: Central-acting drugs are not widely used in initial treatment of high blood pressure but are given along with a diuretic or other antihypertensive drug; peripheral inhibitors, although among the least expensive drugs, tend to cause drowsiness; alpha blockers are usually used in combination with other antihypertensive drugs.

Possible side effects: Orthostatic hypotension (dizziness when patient stands up), nausea, headache, palpitation, impotence, nightmares, loss of appetite, rash, joint pains, shortness of breath.

Generic and trade names: Doxaosin (Cardura), prazosin (Minipress), clonidine (Catapres), guanabenz (Wytensin), reserpine (Serpasil).

Successful Drug Therapy

The alphabet soup of cardiovascular drugs probably seems indecipherable and overwhelming. Each group of drugs has its own set of special considerations and rather daunting list of possible side effects. Indeed, finding the right drug, or combination of drugs, to provide you with symptomatic relief with few or no side effects is not always an easy task.

Like any other drugs, those that treat hypertension and/or heart disease will affect your body in a number of different ways, and it's up to you to learn as much as you can about both the benefits and the drawbacks of drug therapy and consult closely with your physician. When you first start taking your medication, you should plan to see your physician often, perhaps on a weekly or a biweekly basis for a month or so in order to fine-tune treatment.

You should tell your doctor *every* side effect you have; don't worry how major or minor it seems. Any number of alternate therapies may be available to you if one drug or drug combination makes you feel uncomfortable. No matter how unpleasant or embarrassing to you a side effect is, you must never stop taking a drug without first discussing it with your physician.

Doug J., a thirty-eight-year-old patient of mine taking a diuretic to treat high blood pressure and a nitrate for angina, suffered silently for months with headaches and impotence. He thought, as probably most of us would, that he was having severe headaches because he was frustrated at being unable to perform sexually. In fact, both of his problems were caused by the kinds of drugs he was taking. After a few adjustments, Doug felt like his old self again.

Other tips for managing your cardiovascular disease therapy include:

Reduce other risk factors for cardiovascular disease. Stop smoking, avoid excess salt and fat intake, lose weight if you're overweight, and exercise regularly.

Take your medications faithfully. It is imperative to your health that you take your medicine exactly how and when it is prescribed to you in a consistent manner.

Never increase, decrease, stop, or start your medications without your doctor's permission. Doing so could be extremely dangerous. Contact your doctor if you think your medication should be changed.

Let all physicians who treat you know you are taking cardiovascular medication. If you are being treated for any other condition by a doctor other than the one who treats your hypertension and/or heart disease, make sure your physicians communicate with one another. If another doctor changes your blood pressure medication for any reason, ask him or her to send a letter to your primary doctor explaining the change that was made and why it was made. Ask that copies of any blood tests, x-rays, or EKGs be sent to the physician who is treating your cardiovascular disease. If you are hospitalized for any reason, be sure that the doctor treating you for hypertension is informed immediately. Do not rely on another doctor or nurse to do this; they often forget!

Monitor your blood pressure often. Take advantage of every opportunity to have your blood pressure measured by a health care professional; record all blood pressure measurements and bring them to your next appointment.

Make sure you have an ample supply of your medication. If you suddenly stop taking your medication—particularly antihypertensive medication—you will put your health, even your life, at risk. Be sure to ask for new prescriptions at your office visits to avoid running out of pills.

SURGICAL MANAGEMENT OF CORONARY HEART DISEASE

So far, you've read about two ways to treat coronary artery disease: reducing risk factors such as hypertension, obesity, and smoking and/or taking medication designed to lower blood pressure, lower blood cholesterol, or control anginal symptoms. A third option—surgery or angioplasty—is available when these methods have failed or if the disease is sufficiently advanced as to warrant immediate attention.

As you know, coronary heart disease is caused by atherosclerosis: the buildup of plaque deposits containing cholesterol, connective tissue, and calcium that intrude into the vessels, thus reducing the amount of blood delivered to the heart muscle. Surgery to correct this condition involves either widening the vessel by lessening the intrusion of plaque (called angioplasty) or by creating a new route for blood flow that circumvents the blocked part of the artery (called coronary artery bypass).

These surgical techniques are among the most common procedures performed in the United States today. In fact, some studies have shown that they are *over*performed, that many patients undergo unnecessary angioplasties or bypass operations. However, it remains true that blacks are less likely to undergo these procedures than our white counterparts, due largely to the lack of quality health care among the black population and a general fear of the medical establishment by black patients and, in part, to racial discrimination.

If your physician recommends one of these procedures to you, make sure you know exactly why he or she feels it is necessary before you agree. Although both operations are relatively safe, they are costly and entail some risk to you. That said, they can provide relief from the symptoms of heart disease, specifically the often debilitating angina pectoris and the risk of a first or subsequent heart attack. Choosing which procedure is indicated involves a number of different factors, including how many and which heart vessels are involved and the state of your overall health. It is a decision you must reach in close consultation with your physician.

Balloon Angioplasty

As its name implies, balloon angioplasty uses a miniature balloon that when inflated inside a coronary artery compresses plaques against the artery's walls, thereby widening the route of blood flow. It is an extremely common procedure—more than 225,000 are performed every year—and involves minimal risks to the patient. Unlike coronary bypass surgery, angioplasty usually requires a local rather than a general anesthetic and involves minimal recovery time.

An angioplasty is performed in a catheterization laboratory that resembles a hospital operating room. The patient lies flat on a table and is given a local anesthetic. A needle puncture is then made in the patient's groin to gain access to the femoral artery, a vessel that leads to the heart. A guidewire is then threaded through the artery up into the affected coronary vessel; the cardiologist is able to monitor the position of the wire through an x-ray or ultrasound imaging.

Once the guidewire reaches the area where the vessel is blocked by plaque, a balloon catheter is threaded over the guidewire until the balloon is positioned at the site of the blockage. The balloon is inflated, allowed to remain inflated for a few minutes, then deflated. This process is repeated from one to six or seven times. Each time the balloon is inflated, it presses against the plaque, causing it to compress against the vessel wall and split. The heart then should receive adequate blood flow from that artery. Once the artery has thus been widened, the catheter and the guidewire are withdrawn and pressure is applied to the site of the needle puncture for about twenty minutes to prevent bleeding. If all goes smoothly, the patient should be able to leave the hospital the next day.

Although angioplasty is considered a safe and effective procedure—more than 90 percent of patients experience relief of angina—it is not without risks. In about 4 percent of all cases, the artery involved will go into spasm, is split by the catheter, or is blocked by a blood clot. At this point, the physician will attempt to reinflate the balloon to reopen the artery. But if this fails, or the artery closes after the angioplasty has been completed, emergency bypass surgery may be needed.

One of the major drawbacks of angioplasty is that about a third of all angioplasty patients will experience reblockage of the vessel within about six months. It also must be stressed that angioplasty does not *cure* coronary heart disease: what has caused your heart to become damaged is the buildup of fatty plaques. Unless the amount of fat in your bloodstream is lowered, it is likely that reblockage will occur.

Coronary Bypass Grafting

Coronary bypass surgery is an open heart procedure, which means it involves the opening of the chest wall and exposure of the heart. It takes several hours, involves general anesthesia, and requires several weeks of recuperation. Despite these drawbacks, bypass surgery is relatively safe and extremely common: more than 320,000 people undergo the procedure every year. During coronary bypass surgery, the heart must be stopped for the duration of the procedure and its function taken over by a heart-lung machine. This machine captures deoxygenated blood before it enters the heart, oxygenates, filters, and cools it, then returns it to the aorta where it is pumped into general circulation.

Bypass surgery involves taking a vessel from another part of the body—usually the saphenous vein from the leg or an internal mammary artery from the chest—and grafting it onto the heart. The new vessel connects the aorta with the coronary artery beyond the points of blockage, thereby allowing increased amounts of freshly oxygenated blood to areas of the heart that were previously oxygen-starved (Figure 5). In many cases, more than one of the patient's three coronary arteries are blocked. In those instances, more than one vessel is grafted onto the heart in procedures known as double or triple bypass.

Once the operation is completed, the heart is restarted, the heart-lung machine disconnected, and the patient's chest cavity closed. Recovery from bypass surgery usually involves a hospital stay of one to two weeks, followed by several weeks of recuperation at home during which normal activity is gradually resumed. As is the case with angioplasty, coronary artery bypass may not solve the

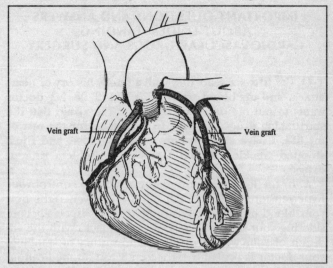

Figure 5 Coronary bypass surgery involves grafting new vessels that literally bypass blocked coronary arteries to bring oxygenated blood to heart tissue.

problem completely or permanently. In fact, some patients find that within just a month or two another occlusion has occurred, requiring another bypass operation.

Indeed, although both angioplasty and coronary artery bypass provide patients with relief from symptoms and may indeed help to prevent a heart attack from occurring, they are not cures. To be effective, these procedures must be paired with major lifestyle changes to reduce the conditions that caused the heart disease to occur in the first place.

Despite your best efforts, and the best efforts of your doctor, you may find yourself among the more than 1 million people who suffer a heart attack every year. In the next chapter, you'll find out what happens during a heart attack, how to prepare yourself for a medical emergency, and how good life can be even after a heart attack occurs.

IMPORTANT QUESTIONS AND ANSWERS ABOUT UNDERSTANDING CARDIOVASCULAR DRUGS AND SURGERY

Q. I'm fifty-six years old, with a family history of heart attack, and my blood pressure is at 172/98. My doctor wants to put me on medication, but I'm afraid that if I start taking drugs, I'll have to take them for the rest of my life. I have about twenty pounds to lose, and I just stopped smoking. Could I solve my problem without drugs?

A. In the long run, you might be able to control your hypertension without medication. However, right now your blood pressure needs to be treated, especially considering your family history of heart attack. With the addition of your weight problem and history of smoking, your doctor is probably right to put you on medication. However, it is quite possible that once your blood pressure is controlled and you've lost the weight, your doctor may slowly wean you from the antihypertensive medication. However, *do not* stop taking your medication without first consulting your physician.

Q. I'm a thirty-six-year-old new mother with high blood pressure. I want to nurse, but am afraid the drugs I've been prescribed will harm my baby. Are there any high blood pressure medicines that I can use?

A. This is an important question, since almost every medicine enters breast milk to some degree. Some drugs enter the breast milk freely, others in very limited amounts. Request that your obstetrician/gynecologist consult with your primary physician about what treatment is best for you and your baby.

CHAPTER 9

Understanding Heart Attacks and Their Aftermath

"I know it sounds like a cliché, but it felt like a truck was on my chest and someone was squeezing my heart like a lemon," recalls Thomas K., the paralegal you met in Chapter 5. "For a good hour, I thought it was just indigestion, although I was pale and sweating. And really, I would have waited even longer before doing anything about it, but a colleague of mine took one look at me and figured I was having a heart attack. He made me go to the hospital."

Thomas was indeed having a heart attack. A blood clot called a thrombus had blocked off one coronary artery, an artery that had already been narrowed by atherosclerosis. The part of his heart fed by that artery was dying from lack of oxygen, and the pain of that death was radiating through his body. The longer Thomas waited, the more damage the blockage would do to his heart.

When Thomas arrived at the emergency room, he was immediately examined by a physician, placed on oxygen, given an EKG, and a needle was inserted in his arm to provide access to intravenous medication. He was given an aspirin, a nitroglycerin tablet to reduce the pain, and probably a beta blocker. At the same time, a series of blood tests were performed. When the EKG results revealed that he was indeed suffering from a heart attack, thrombolytic drugs—highly effective drugs to break up blood clots—were administered. When administered within six hours of the onset of a heart attack, thrombolytic agents dissolve blood clots and restore blood flow to the heart in more than two-thirds of heart attack cases.

If Thomas's heartbeat had remained dangerously unstable ninety minutes after the thrombolytic agents were administered, cardiac angioplasty—the placement of a balloon pump to widen the coronary arteries—may have been attempted. If his heart had continued to fail, defibrillation (the passage of electricity through the heart to restore normal rhythm) would have been applied. If his heart had stopped completely, cardiopulmonary resuscitation would have been performed. Fortunately he was in stable condition, and those measures were not required.

Nonetheless, Thomas remained under observation in the hospital. A few days later, he was given a stress test—his heart rate was measured by an EKG while he walked on a treadmill—that showed his heart was not receiving enough oxygen. He was then given an angiogram, a procedure in which a blood vessel is filled with a special dye, then x-rayed to identify exactly where a blockage is located. Thomas's physicians decided to schedule him for a balloon angioplasty the next day. As you may remember from Chapter 8, this procedure reduces the impact of atherosclerosis by compressing plaques against artery walls, thereby enabling more blood to reach the heart and lessening the chances that another heart attack would take place.

Thomas remained in the hospital under close observation for another few days, was given another stress test that showed a significant increase in the amount of oxygen his heart was receiving, and was released with orders from me to take it easy and gradually return to his full range of activities. I prescribed small doses of aspirin to be taken on a daily basis and a beta blocker to assist in controlling his blood pressure. Thomas and I also discussed the underlying causes of his cardiovascular disease, including the damage that stress caused by racism in the workplace was doing to his heart and blood vessels, as well as the fact that he was ten pounds overweight and rarely exercised. By the time he left the hospital, Thomas knew that treatment for his heart attack would be a lifelong proposition.

HEART ATTACKS AND AFRICAN-AMERICANS

Thomas K. is a lucky man, first because he was relatively healthy at the time of his heart attack; his heart disease was serious, but clearly not fatal. Thomas is also lucky because he is educated, self-confident, and fully employed with comprehensive health insurance. When he arrived at the hospital, he was treated as every man and woman should be—professionally, quickly, and without regard to his skin color.

Unfortunately, not every black person is so treated, either due to racism or socioeconomic factors. A colleague told me of a thirty-year-old man who came into the emergency room complaining of crushing chest pain. Since he was so young, the emergency room doctors didn't even consider that he might be having a heart attack and were about to discharge him with advice to take an antacid to relieve "indigestion." Luckily, another physician, an African-American woman, thought to ask about his family and personal medical histories before writing him off as a simple case of indigestion. As it turned out, this young man had diabetes and high blood pressure, and both his father and brother had had heart attacks at early ages. The physician ordered the routine tests and determined that he was indeed having a heart attack.

In my opinion, this case showed at least two discrepancies between the health care received by black and white patients. First, the admitting physicians were careless in their treatment of the patient, perhaps because of racial discrimination, perhaps because they simply didn't know that black patients have higher rates of cardiovascular disease at younger ages than whites.

Second, the black population in general is less educated about cardiovascular disease than the white population. As pointed out in Chapter 1, black heart attack victims are less likely to recognize their symptoms as those of a heart attack than are whites, and they are much more likely to ascribe them to something else, like heartburn or indigestion. The same lack of education about risk factors for cardiovascular disease—like diabetes, obesity, and a family history of heart attacks—no doubt contributes to the higher rate of fatal heart attacks in this population.

The fact that you are reading this book means that this lack of education may soon become a thing of the past. By taking the time to learn about your risks of a heart attack, how to protect yourself from them, and what to do if one occurs, you are taking control of your health in a very positive way.

The Medical Emergency

As you may remember from Chapter 2, coronary artery disease involves fatty deposits called plaque, which build up on the walls of the arteries that feed the heart muscle. When blood flow is reduced to the point where the heart muscle cannot get enough oxygen, a condition known as myocardial ischemia may result. With ischemia, some oxygen still reaches the heart, but the supply is diminished. Symptoms of ischemia include angina (chest pain) and shortness of breath. Angina attacks usually occur during periods of intense activity or stress and resolve themselves within thirty minutes.

A heart attack, on the other hand, involves the actual death of heart tissue and the symptoms are usually

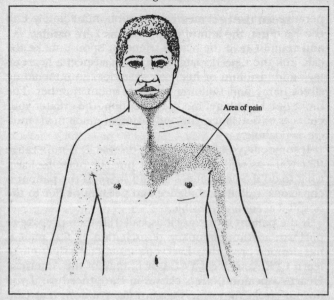

Area of pain

Figure 6   Unlike myocardial ischemia (narrowing), a myocardial infarction, or heart attack, involves complete blockage of one of the three coronary arteries. This blockage keeps heart tissue from receiving the oxygen it needs to survive.

longer lasting and more severe than those that accompany angina (Figure 6). Like Thomas K., a person having a heart attack will experience a crushing pressure or burning sensation in the chest. This pain may radiate to the shoulders or arms—usually on the left side—or to the neck, jaw, or back. The heart attack victim may also feel dizzy, nauseated, or faint.

In certain cases, the lack of oxygen will cause the heart to stop completely, a condition known as cardiac arrest. If the heart action and circulation are not returned within just a few moments, the chance that full recovery will occur is low. This type of sudden death from a heart attack occurs in about 300,000 patients every year.

If you experience symptoms of a heart attack, it is imperative that you get medical attention immediately. Call the Emergency Medical Service (EMS) by dialing 911 and request help, or have a friend or spouse make the call. Tell the EMS dispatcher that you suspect a heart attack and give him or her your exact location, including street name and building and apartment number. The more quickly you get medical attention, the greater your chances of both surviving and saving as much heart muscle as possible.

If someone you love has heart disease, it is imperative that you—as well as the patient him- or herself—learn what to do if a heart attack should strike. If the patient is conscious, call an ambulance and get him or her to the hospital as soon as possible.

If the patient is unconscious, call 911, then prepare to perform cardiopulmonary resuscitation if the patient has stopped breathing. Everyone should take the time to learn CPR; your local YWCA or branch of the American Heart Association offers classes in the procedure if you do not already know it. Please note, however, that CPR can be dangerous if not practiced with care. The instructions in Table 14 will help you better understand the procedure, but it is best for you to learn the correct technique from a trained professional.

The Extent of Heart Damage

When heart tissue dies because a coronary artery has become blocked, several things can occur. If the damaged area is small, full heart function may return on its own—in cases of very mild heart attacks, in fact, the victims may never even realize they have had one. In other cases, however, the damage is more serious.

Cardiac arrhythmias occur when the blockage causes a malfunction of the heart's electrical impulse system, leading to various types of irregular heart rhythms and thus an ineffective pumping of the heart muscle. One particularly serious complication of arrhythmia is ventricular fibrillation, which explains why the emergency

TABLE 14 Cardiopulmonary Resuscitation (CPR)

1. *Attempt to rouse the victim.* Gently shake the victim by the shoulders and shout "Are you okay?" several times. If the patient does not respond, call for help, then check to see if he or she is breathing.

2. *Lay the victim on his or her back.* For CPR to be effective, the patient must be lying on his or her back on a firm, flat surface. To turn over someone who is facedown, first take the arm closest to you and stretch it out straight behind his or her head. With one hand behind the victim's neck for support, grasp the arm farthest from you above the elbow and roll the victim toward you.

3. *Open his or her airway.* If the patient is unable to breathe, it is important that you open his or her airway, which may be blocked by the tongue. Place one hand on the victim's forehead and place the middle fingers of the other hand on the victim's jaw. Push down on the forehead while lifting the chin up. This will lift the tongue away from the back of the throat.

4. *Check for breathing.* While maintaining the tilted position of the head, place your ear over the victim's mouth and listen for breathing sounds; check to see if the chest is rising and falling; see if you can feel the victim's breath on your cheek by holding your face near his or her mouth and nose. If the victim is breathing, wait for medical help. If not, go on to next step.

5. *Start mouth-to-mouth breathing.* Still maintaining the victim's head position, use the thumb and forefinger of one hand to pinch closed the victim's nose to keep air from escaping. Take a deep breath, open your mouth wide, and place your lips around the outside of the victim's mouth. Exhale forcefully, then remove your mouth. Repeat the procedure. If this has not reestablished respiration, go on to next step.

6. *Check for a pulse.* Place two fingers of one hand (not your thumb) to the side of the victim's throat (next to the Adam's apple). If you can feel a pulse, cardiac arrest has not occurred—the heart is still pumping blood to the brain and the rest of the body. If this is the case, but the patient is still not breathing, continue mouth-to-mouth resuscitation. If the victim does not have a pulse, you must attempt to restart the heart.

7. *Perform a chest thump.* Gently lower the victim's head to the floor. You make a fist with one hand, closing the thumb inside. Strike the victim in the middle of his or her chest with a strong thump; if the heart does not start, begin chest compressions.

8. *Begin chest compressions.* Kneel at right angles to the victim with your knees at about his or her shoulders. With one hand, try to find the sternum, the spot near the center of the chest where the ribs meet the breastbone. Place the heel of your hand on the sternum and place your other hand on top of it. Shift your weight forward, and keeping your elbows locked, push down one to two inches for about a half a second and come up again. Do this fifteen times, then give the patient two mouth-to-mouth breaths. Repeat the cycle of fifteen compressions and two mouth breaths four times—this should take about one minute—then take the victim's pulse again. Continue until the patient has resumed consciousness, the EMS team has arrived, or until you are too exhausted to continue.

team working on Thomas K. was ready to defibrillate his heart with drugs or electric shock therapy. If the normal heart rate and rhythm are not restored, cardiac arrest, complete failure of the heart muscle to pump, can occur, and is often fatal. In cases of chronic cardiac arrhythmias, one of several types of artificial devices that restore normal heart rate may be implanted in the heart or chest.

Heart failure, otherwise known as congestive heart failure, is a condition in which the heart keeps pumping, but does so inefficiently because it has been damaged. Because the heart does not pump a normal amount of blood into the arterial circulation, pressure can build up in the venous circulation. This may cause congestion—buildup of fluids—in various organs, including the lungs and liver. Heart failure is usually treated with one or more cardiovascular drugs to lower blood pressure and reduce the action of the heart.

When the heart becomes too damaged to function, a heart transplant may be indicated. In this major surgery, a healthy heart harvested from a recently deceased donor is placed in the patient's chest after his or her own diseased organ has been removed. Although transplants are largely successful, they require patients to take strong drugs, called immunosuppressants, for the rest of their lives. These drugs, which suppress the immune system so that the new heart will not be rejected by the body, may have serious side effects, especially with long-term use. In addition, the procedure remains expensive and organ donors remain scarce, making the operation viable only as a last resort.

Life After a Heart Attack

Heart attack survivors who show no signs of heart failure or arrhythmias within two or three days following their attack are likely to fully recover and are often discharged from the hospital within a week or two. Like Thomas K., they may require angioplasty, bypass surgery, and/or drug therapy to ensure that sufficient blood flow to the heart continues. Although the time it takes to fully recover varies from patient to patient, most survivors find they can return to their normal routines—including work, exercise, and sexual relations—within several weeks.

For most people, a heart attack marks an important turning point in their lives. Although some resign themselves to lifelong illness, most are inspired by their survival of this medical crisis. They regard it as an opportunity to make healthy changes in their lives and in the lives of those they love. The changes involve reducing the very same risk factors that caused the heart attack to occur: stopping smoking and other substance abuse, reducing stress, lowering salt and fat intake, and incorporating exercise into their everyday lives.

I hope this book has inspired you to reduce your risk of developing hypertension and heart disease in time to prevent a first—or even a second or third—heart attack. It's never too late for you or your family to change those habits that are damaging to your health and to live life with renewed vigor and strength. Indeed, it's never too late for you to take control!

IMPORTANT QUESTIONS AND ANSWERS ABOUT UNDERSTANDING HEART ATTACK AND ITS AFTERMATH

Q. I've been told that I have coronary heart disease and am at risk for a heart attack. I've learned the symptoms of a heart attack and know how to get help quickly. Does that mean I'll survive a heart attack if I have one?

A. By learning the symptoms of heart attack, you've significantly increased the odds not only that you'll survive, but that the damage to your heart will be limited. However, there are no guarantees. Much depends on which of your three coronary arteries become blocked and what part of the heart muscle is damaged. In less than a third of all heart attacks, the heart attack causes so much damage in such a short amount of time that death occurs within just a few moments.

You can further increase your odds of survival—and of having a heart attack in the first place—by reducing your blood pressure, cutting down on the fats you eat, and getting plenty of exercise.

Q. My father had a heart attack. We thought he was going to be fine, but the next day, while he was still in intensive care, he had a stroke that has completely disabled him. Were the two events connected?

A. Probably. What happened to your father happens to some degree to about 10 percent of all heart attack victims. An embolus, a blood clot, breaks off from the damaged heart vessel and travels through the bloodstream until it reaches a vessel in the brain too narrow to allow it to pass. The resulting blockage keeps oxygen-rich blood from reaching part of the brain, causing the stroke.

Q. My wife has had a heart attack and now I'm afraid that if we have sex, she'll have another one. Is it possible?

A. Although sexual intercourse will raise your wife's blood pressure and pulse rate, unless her heart is severely damaged, she should be able to tolerate the stress. However, to be sure, your wife should ask her physician to perform a stress test on her to measure how her heart is functioning.

Resources

YOUR HEART AND CIRCULATORY SYSTEM

General information on prevention and treatment of cardiovascular disease is available from the organizations listed below. In addition, should you want to learn more about CPR and other emergency care procedures, the Red Cross offers classes in many communities. The American Heart Association, with branches in every major city across the country, provides pamphlets, videotapes, and classes on all aspects of cardiovascular disease, including diet and exercise plans to lower the risks of hypertension and heart disease, the latest research on medical breakthroughs, and pamphlets on symptoms of heart attacks, strokes, and other cardiovascular emergencies.

The American Heart Association
7320 Greenville Avenue
Dallas, TX 75231
(214) 373-6300
(800) 553-6321
Web site: www.americanheart.org

American Red Cross
430 17th Street NW
Washington, DC 20006
Web site: www.usa.redcross.org

Office of Disease Prevention and Health Promotion
National Health Information Center
P.O. Box 1133
Washington, DC 20013-11332
(800) 336-4797
Web site: www.nhic-nt.health.org

National Heart, Lung, and Blood Institute
National Institutes of Health
9000 Rockville Pike
Building 31, Room 4A-21
Bethesda, MD 20892
(301) 496-4236
Web site: www.nhlbi.gov

National High Blood Pressure Education Program
Information Center
National Institutes of Health
9000 Rockville Pike, Building 31 Suite 4A-16
Bethesda, MD 20814
(301) 951-3260

PHYSICAL FITNESS AND REHABILITATION

Physical fitness is more than a fad—it's a key ingredient in a healthy life. In almost every neighborhood,
health clubs and spas, not to mention the old reliable
YMCA, can get you in shape in just a few months of hard
work. If you've had a heart attack, however, you may
need special help. The following organizations will help
you find resources near your home:

National Rehabilitation Association
1910 Association Drive
Reston, VA 22091
(703) 715-9090

National Rehabilitation Information Center
8455 Colesville Road
Silver Spring, MD 20910
(301) 588-9284
(800) 346-2742

SMOKING, CARDIOVASCULAR DISEASE, AND CANCER

Many people need encouragement and help to stop smoking. The organizations listed below can give you advice on how to stop smoking on your own or recommend reputable medical or psychological techniques:

Minority Outreach Initiative
American Lung Association
1740 Broadway
New York, NY 10019
(212) 315-8700
(800) 586-4872

National Center for Health Promotion
Smoker Stoppers Program
3920 Varsity Drive
Ann Arbor, MI 48108
(313) 971-6077

Smokenders
1430 East Indian School Road
Phoenix, AZ 85014
(800) 828-4357

American Cancer Society
National Office
1599 Clifton Road NE
Atlanta, GA 30329
(404) 320-3333
(800) 227-2345 for all areas of the U.S. except:
Alaska: (800) 638-6070
Hawaii: (800) 524-1234
Web site: www.cancer.org

DRUG ABUSE

Taking drugs puts an individual at risk not only for cardiovascular disease and sudden death, but for a variety of other deadly conditions. For more information about drug abuse and treatment, contact the following organizations:

Drug Abuse and Narcotic Addiction
Cocaine Abuse Hotline
800-COCAINE

Drug Abuse Clearinghouse
P.O. Box 2345
11426 Rockville Pike
Rockville, MD 20852
(301) 443-6500

Drug Crisis Hotline
(800) 522-5353

ALCOHOL ABUSE

Heavy drinking is known to cause myriad physical and emotional problems, including hypertension and heart disease. If you think you or someone you love has a problem with alcohol, contact the following organizations:

1-800-ALCOHOL (24-hour hotline)

Alcoholics Anonymous, Inc.
15 East 26th Street
New York, NY 10010
(212) 683-3900

DIABETES

Diabetes is epidemic among the black population, and often coexists with cardiovascular disease. Combined with smoking, hypertension, atherosclerosis, and a sedentary lifestyle, diabetes is a leading risk factor in the development of heart attacks and stroke. For more information on treatment for diabetes, contact:

American Diabetes Association, Inc.
16600 Duke Street
Alexandria, VA 22314
(800) 342-2383
Web site: www.diabetes.com

National Diabetes Information Clearinghouse
National Institutes of Health
Box NDIC
9000 Rockville Pike
Bethesda, MD 20892
(301) 468-2162

KIDNEY DISEASE

Damage to the kidneys is both a cause and effect of high blood pressure. The National Kidney Foundation is an excellent source of general information about all aspects of kidney disease. For patients who have specific kidney problems and want to learn more about support groups for kidney patients or receive the quarterly publication *Renal Life,* written by and for those with kidney disorders, contact the American Association of Kidney Patients.

American Association of Kidney Patients
1 Davis Boulevard, Suite LLI
Tampa, FL 33606
(813) 251-0725

National Kidney Foundation
30 East 33rd Street
New York, NY 10016
(212) 889-2210

NUTRITION EDUCATION

What you eat has an enormous impact on the health of your heart and circulatory system. It is essential that you lower the amount of salt and fat in your diet if you want to avoid cardiovascular disease. In addition to the American Heart Association (listed above), the following organizations can provide you with nutrition information:

American Dietetic Association
216 West Jackson
Chicago, IL 60606
(312) 899-0040

National Cholesterol Education Program
National Institutes of Health
9000 Rockville Pike
Building 31, Suite 4A-16
Bethesda, MD 20814

STROKE AND ITS AFTERMATH

For further information about stroke prevention and treatment, the National Stroke Association, located in Denver, Colorado, has an extensive list of publications and videos. Write to them for a publications list, as well as for information about stroke support groups across the country. The American Heart Association is another excellent source of information on this subject.

The National Stroke Association
96 Inverness Drive, Suite I
Englewood, CO 80112
1-800-STROKES (1-800-787-6537)

Glossary

Aerobic Exercise: Physical exercise that relies on oxygen for energy production.

Adrenal Glands: Hormone-producing (endocrine) glands, located on top of each kidney, responsible for secreting several hormones related to blood pressure, including adrenaline and aldosterone.

Aldosterone: A steroid hormone that is released by the adrenal gland and acts on the kidneys to promote conservation of sodium and water, thereby raising blood pressure.

Aneurism: A bulging, weak portion of a blood vessel.

Angiogram: A diagnostic x-ray of blood vessels or other parts of the circulatory system. The procedure involves injecting dye into the bloodstream to make blood vessels or the heart visible on an x-ray.

Angioplasty: A therapeutic procedure in which a catheter with a deflated balloon at the tip is inserted into an artery blocked by atherosclerotic plaque. When the balloon is inflated, it splits the plaque open, thereby increasing blood flow.

Angiotensin/Angiotensin II: Substances in the blood produced in response to release by the kidneys of the enzyme renin. Angiotensin is an important vasoconstrictor, or substance that raises blood pressure by narrowing the blood vessels. Angiotensin also causes an increase in the output of aldosterone.

Aorta: The largest artery in the body, from which all others branch. The main vessel leading away from the heart, which receives blood from the left ventricle of the heart.

Arrhythmia: Irregular heartbeat.

Arteries: Blood vessels that carry oxygenated blood away from the heart to nourish cells throughout the body.

Arterioles: Small arterial vessels most responsible for the control of blood pressure. They pass blood from the arteries to the capillaries.

Arteriogram: An examination of a portion of the circulatory system performed by injecting dye into the artery, thereby forming a map of the vessels that can be examined by x-ray.

Aspirin (acetylsalicylic acid): A drug that reduces inflammation and fever. It is also known to affect the platelets in the blood to prevent thickening or clotting.

Atherosclerosis: A disease of the arteries in which fatty plaques develop on the inner walls.

Atrial Fibrillation: An abnormal heart rhythm in which the heart's atria contract too fast and at an irregular rate.

Atrium: An upper chamber of the heart. There are two atria.

Autonomic Nervous System: The involuntary nervous system responsible for bodily functions such as heartbeat, blood pressure, digestion, etc. It is divided into two separate divisions, the sympathetic nervous system and the parasympathetic nervous system.

Biofeedback: A behavior modification therapy in which patients are taught to control usually unconscious bodily functions, such as blood pressure, through conscious effort. In addition, biofeedback is used as a stroke rehabilitation method.

Blood Vessels: Tubes of smooth muscle that carry blood from and to the heart. Arteries and veins are the two main types of blood vessels.

Calorie: A basic unit of energy measurement; 1 calorie is the amount of heat required to raise the temperature of 1 gram of water by 1 degree Centigrade.

Capillaries: The smallest of the blood vessels, they form networks in most tissues. Supplied with blood by arterioles, the capillaries have walls just one cell thick, which allow fluids, oxygen, and other nutrients to pass.

Carbohydrate: Organic compounds of carbon, hydrogen, and oxygen, which include starches, cellulose, and sugars, and are an important source of energy. All carbohydrates are eventually broken down in the body to glucose, a simple sugar. Excess carbohydrates are stored as fats in the liver and muscles.

Cardiac Arrest: An incident in which the heart stops beating.

Cardiac Catheterization: A diagnostic exam in which a catheter is inserted through the blood vessels into the chambers of the heart.

Cardiopulmonary Resuscitation: A lifesaving procedure for a person suffering cardiac arrest involving compression of the heart muscle and mouth-to-mouth breathing to restore blood circulation to the brain.

Cardiovascular System: The heart together with the two networks of blood vessels—arteries and veins—that transport nutrients and oxygen to the tissues and remove waste products.

Central Nervous System: The brain and the spinal cord, which are responsible for the integration of all nervous activities.

Cholesterol: A fatlike substance found in the brain, nerves, liver, blood, and bile. Synthesized in the liver, cholesterol is essential in a number of bodily functions. Excess consumption of dietary cholesterol, found in animal products, such as red meat, whole milk, and eggs, contributes to atherosclerosis and coronary heart disease.

Coronary Arteries: The two main vessels that supply the heart with blood.

Coronary Bypass Surgery: Surgery to improve blood

flow to the heart, involving the grafting of a blood vessel taken from the leg or chest around the blocked section of the aortic artery.

Coronary Heart Disease: Diseases of the heart caused by a narrowing of the coronary arteries, resulting in reduced blood flow to the heart.

Diabetes Mellitus: A chronic illness characterized by an excess of blood sugar, which is due either to insufficient insulin production in the pancreas or the inability of the body to use insulin properly. Long-term effects of diabetes include increased risk for atherosclerosis and vision problems.

Diastole: The interval between heartbeats when the heart relaxes and fills with blood. The diastolic reading in a blood pressure measurement is the lower number.

Diuretic: A type of antihypertension drug that works to lower blood pressure by promoting salt and water excretion, which lowers the volume of the blood.

Echocardiography: Diagnostic procedure that uses ultrasound waves to visualize structures within the heart.

Electrocardiography (EKG or ECG): A procedure in which heart function is measured by the tracing of its electrical impulses.

Embolism: Obstruction of a blood vessel by a foreign body (a blood clot, a clot of fat, or an air bubble) that has moved through the bloodstream from its point of origin to a narrower branch of the vessel. The material causing the blockage is called an embolus.

Epinephrine: Also called adrenaline. A hormone secreted by the adrenal glands, situated just above the kidneys, that increases the heart rate and constricts blood vessels.

Essential Hypertension: High blood pressure caused by an unknown factor or factors. Accounts for approximately 90 percent of hypertension cases.

Fat: An essential nutrient, the principal form in which energy is stored in the body.

Fibrillation: Uncoordinated tremors of the heart resulting in an irregular pulse.

Fight-or-Flight Response: The body's response to perceived danger or stress, involving the release of hormones and subsequent rise in heart rate, blood pressure, and muscle tension.

Glucose: The most common simple sugar; the essential source of energy for the body. It is stored in the liver as glycogen but can be converted back into glucose rapidly.

Heart Attack: The death of heart tissue caused by interruption of the blood circulation through the coronary arteries. Also called myocardial infarction.

Heart Failure: A condition in which the heart muscle is unable to pump enough blood to maintain normal circulation; this results in a buildup of fluid in the body. Also called congestive heart failure.

Heart Rate: The number of times the heart beats (contracts) per minute.

Hemoglobin: The oxygen-carrying red pigment component of the red blood cells. Hemoglobin transports oxygen to the body tissue and removes carbon dioxide.

Hemorrhage: Bleeding due to the rupture of a blood vessel.

High-Density Lipoprotein: A lipid-carrying protein that transports the so-called good cholesterol away from the artery walls to the liver.

Hyperlipidemia: Excessive fats in the blood.

Hypertension: High blood pressure.

Hypokalemia: A depletion of potassium in the blood, which is a side effect of some antihypertension drugs.

Hypotension: Low blood pressure.

Infarction: The death of tissue that occurs when the blood supply to a localized part of the body is blocked.

Ischemia: Oxygen deficiency caused by an obstruction of the blood vessel.

Kidneys: The two bean-shaped glands, situated at the back of the abdomen, that regulate salt, volume, and composition of body fluids by filtering the blood and eliminating waste through the production of urine.

Lipids: Fats, steroids, phospholipids, and glycolipids; fat or fatlike substances.

Lipoprotein: Responsible for the transport of lipids in the blood and body fluid.

Low-Density Lipoprotein: The lipid-carrying protein that transports the so-called bad cholesterol into the bloodstream.

Myocardial Infarction: *See* Heart attack.

Nicotine: A poisonous substance derived from tobacco. Tobacco smoke elevates blood pressure and pulse rate.

Norepinephrine: Also called noradrenaline. A hormone secreted by the adrenal gland that raises blood pressure by constricting small blood vessels and increasing blood flow through the coronary arteries.

Obesity: The condition in which excess fat has accumulated in the body. Usually considered to be present when a person is 20 percent above the recommended weight for his or her height.

Plaque: Fatty deposits that build up on the inner walls of the blood vessels, thereby obstructing the normal flow of blood.

Platelet: Component of the blood most specifically involved in blood clotting.

Polyunsaturated Fats: A type of fat derived from plants, such as vegetables, that does not elevate blood cholesterol levels.

Renal Arteries: The two large arteries that supply blood to the kidney.

Renin: An enzyme found in the kidney that is transformed by other body tissues into angiotensin, which raises blood pressure in response to stress.

Risk Factor: Condition or behavior that increases one's likelihood of developing a disease or injury.

Saturated Fats: A type of fat derived mainly from animal products that causes an elevation in blood cholesterol levels.

Sclerosis: An abnormal thickening or hardening of the arteries and other vessels.

Secondary Hypertension: High blood pressure caused by a specific organ defect or disease.

Smooth Muscle: Under the control of the autonomic

nervous system, muscles that produce long-term, slow contractions, such as those that occur in blood vessels.

Sodium: A mineral found in table salt and essential body constituents. Controls the volume of fluids outside the cells. The amount of sodium in the body is controlled by the kidneys.

Sphygmomanometer: An instrument used to measure blood pressure.

Stress: Any factor that has an adverse effect on the body, physical or emotional.

Stroke: An interruption of the blood flow to the brain.

Sympathetic Nervous System: The division of the autonomic nervous system responsible for reflex actions such as blood pressure, salivation, and digestion.

Systole: The contraction of the heart muscle. Systolic pressure is the greater of the two blood pressure readings.

Tachycardia: Abnormally rapid and irregular heartbeat.

Thrombosis: The formation of a blood clot, called a thrombus, that partially or completely blocks a blood vessel.

Triglyceride: The most common lipid found in fatty tissue; the form in which fat is stored in the body.

Vascular: Pertaining to, or supplied with, vessels, usually blood vessels.

Index

ABOUT THE AUTHORS

PAUL A. JONES, M.D., is Chief Fellow of Cardiovascular Medicine at Loyola University Medical Center, Illinois, and an associate member of the American College of Cardiology. Dr. Jones has taught at the University of Illinois College of Medicine and spent time in private practice.

ANGELA MITCHELL is a free-lance writer, now based in Chicago, Illinois, who has written on medical topics for *Emerge* and the *Village Voice*. Ms. Mitchell graduated from Brown University.

LINDA VILLAROSA, currently science editor at *The New York Times*, is the author of three books, including *Body & Soul: The Black Women's Guide to Physical Health and Emotional Well-Being*. She has also written for *American Health, Mademoiselle, Ms.*, among other national publications.

MAUDENE NELSON, M.S., R.D., a registered dietician and certified diabetes educator, is a staff associate at the Institute of Human Nutrition, College of Physicians & Surgeons, Columbia University, and a nutritionist for the Arteriosclerosis Research at Columbia Presbyterian Medical Center.